# Get Fit Now:

## Your Roadmap to a Healthier, Stronger You

**Table Of Content**

*Part I: Laying the Groundwork*

### 26. **Overcoming Plateaus**
- What to do when your progress stalls.

### 27. **Dealing with Injuries**
- How to handle injuries without derailing your fitness journey.

### 28. **Exercise and Chronic Illness**
- Managing conditions like diabetes and hypertension through fitness.

### 29. **Motivation: Keeping the Fire Alive**
- Strategies to keep yourself motivated.

### 30. **The Role of Community**
- Finding and engaging with a supportive fitness community.

*Part VII: Advanced Topics*

### 31. **High-Intensity Training**
- A look at more intense forms of exercise and their benefits.

### 32. **Periodization: Planning for Long-term Success**
- How to structure your training cycles for optimal gains.

### 33. **Advanced Nutrition for Athletes**
- Tailoring your diet for athletic performance.

### 34. **Biohacking Your Fitness**
- Cutting-edge techniques and technologies to enhance your fitness.

### 35. **Sport-Specific Training**
- How to train for specific sports like swimming, cycling, and running.

*Part VIII: Final Thoughts*

**36. What to Do When You Fall Off the Wagon**
- Strategies for getting back on track.

**37. The Role of Coaching and Mentorship**
- How external guidance can benefit you.

**38. Review and Adjust: Your Evolving Fitness Plan**
- Regularly reviewing and updating your fitness goals and plans.

**39. Case Studies: Real-life Success Stories**
- Testimonials and interviews from people who have successfully improved their fitness.

**40. Conclusion: Your Future in Fitness**
- Wrapping up the book and preparing the reader for a lifelong fitness journey.

# PART I: LAYING THE GROUNDWORK

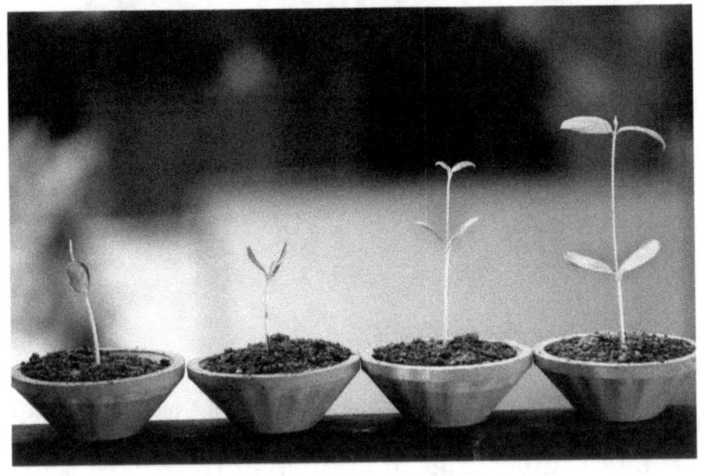

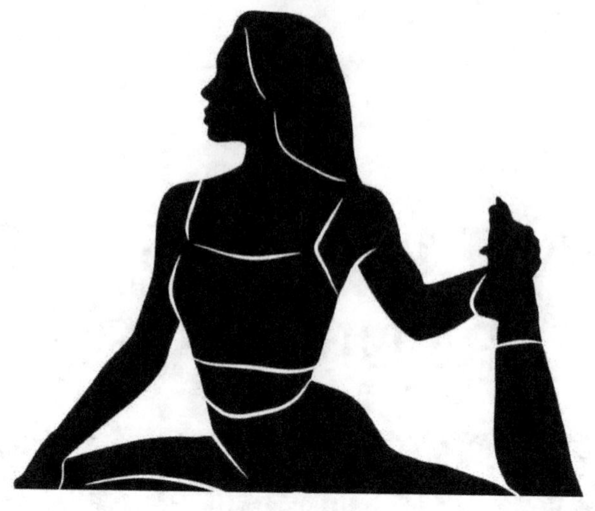

*Chapter 1:*

*Introduction: Your Journey
to Fitness Begins*

## Your Odyssey of Transformation

Welcome to the beginning of the rest of your life. No, that's not hyperbole. Embarking on a journey to fitness will literally change your life—in more ways than you can count. Forget the superficial aspects, like looking good in a bathing suit. Yes, those are perks, but fitness is transformative at a cellular level, shaping not just your body, but your mind, your outlook, and your very essence.

## The Chris Hemsworth Experience

If you've ever marvelled at the sculpted physiques of celebrities like Chris Hemsworth, who underwent a complete transformation to play Thor in the Marvel movies, you might be inspired and intimidated in equal measure.

Yes, Chris had access to the best trainers, dieticians, and a compelling reason to get in shape (a multi-million dollar movie deal is a good motivator), but at its core, his transformation still relied on principles accessible to us all: discipline, dedication, and a commitment to health.

Remember, Chris Hemsworth wasn't born as Thor. He started with an average body but chose to undertake a journey requiring immense dedication. He spent hours at the gym, followed a strict nutrition plan, and did this consistently. His transformation is a loud and clear testament to what is achievable when you set your mind to it.

## What Fitness Really Means

Fitness isn't just about dumbbells and treadmills. It's about enhancing your quality of life. Fitness reduces your risk of chronic illnesses, boosts your mental health, and empowers you to live your life to the fullest.

## The Five Pillars of Fitness

1. **Physical Endurance**: Your ability to sustain long periods of physical activity.

2. **Strength:** The capability of your muscles to lift weight.

3. **Flexibility:** The range of motion around your joints.

4. **Balance:** Your control when you're moving or stationary.

5. **Mental Resilience:** The often-overlooked mental aspect of being fit, including stress management and motivation.

## Daily Tasks and Training Program for the Absolute Beginner

If you're a complete newbie, fear not. We're not going to throw you into the deep end just yet. Instead, we'll start with simple daily tasks and a basic training program to get you acclimated to the fitness lifestyle.

## Daily Tasks

1. **Step Count:** Aim for at least 10,000 steps a day. Use your phone or a pedometer to track this.

2. **Water Intake:** Drink at least 8 cups of water. Start your day with one cup as soon as you wake up.

3. **Meal Planning:** Stick to a balanced meal that includes proteins, healthy fats, and vegetables.

## Basic Training Program (Week 1)

- **Monday**: 20 minutes of brisk walking + 10 body-weight squats

- **Wednesday**: 20 minutes of brisk walking + 10 push-ups (or knee push-ups)

- **Friday**: 20 minutes of brisk walking + 10 body-weight lunges per leg

## Actionable Strategies

1. **Find Your 'Why':** Establish a clear and personal reason for wanting to get fit.

2. **Routine Over Motivation:** You won't always be motivated, but you can always be disciplined. Make fitness a non-negotiable part of your day.

3. **Set Micro-Goals:** Aim for smaller, achievable objectives, like losing 1 pound a week, rather than aiming to lose 50 pounds without a concrete plan.

## Food for Thought

- Is your quest for fitness driven by self-love or self-loathing? The answer can profoundly affect your journey.
- Does your current lifestyle align with the fitness goals you've set? If not, what changes can you implement today?

## Summary

1. **Your Journey Begins:** Fitness isn't merely physical; it impacts every facet of your life.
2. **Learn from the Best:** Even celebrities like Chris Hemsworth start with the basics—dedication and discipline.
3. **The Five Pillars:** Physical endurance, strength, flexibility, balance, and mental resilience make up the holistic view of fitness.
4. **Daily Tasks and Basic Training:** Small, consistent actions can lead to big results.
5. **Actionable Strategies:** Identify your 'Why,' make fitness routine, and set achievable goals to stay on track.

Congratulations, you've just taken the first step on a transformative journey that goes beyond mere aesthetics. In the chapters ahead, we'll explore each element of fitness, nutrition, mental well-being, and much more, in depth. Think of this book as your fitness compass, a tool to guide you as you Explore uncharted territories of your potential. Strap in. It's going to be an exciting journey!

Welcome aboard the fitness train; your life will never be the same!

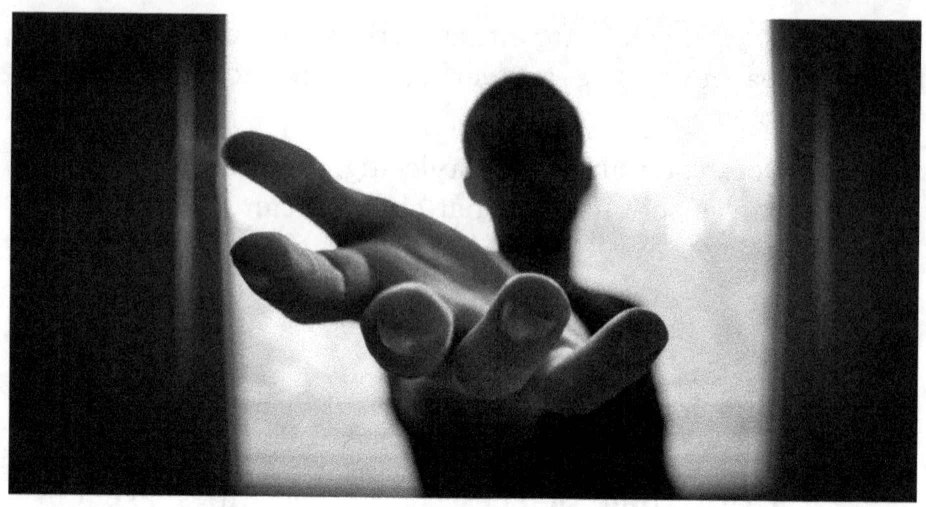

## Chapter 2:

## The Mind-Body Connection: Setting Your Intentions

### Introduction: The Mind as the Rudder

So, you've embarked on your fitness journey. Your running shoes are out of the closet, and your fridge is packed with leafy greens. Great start! But before you break a sweat, let's discuss an often-overlooked cornerstone of your fitness journey: your mind. If the body is a ship, the mind is its rudder. Steering it correctly can make or break your journey to the fabled land of Fitness.

### The Extraordinary Story of Novak Djokovic

Imagine being a professional tennis player diagnosed with a gluten intolerance. It sounds like a career-ending revelation, doesn't it? This was the reality faced by Novak Djokovic. Before 2010, Djokovic was plagued with health issues; he would lose his breath quickly, suffer from frequent injuries, and was unable to maintain peak performance throughout matches. But instead of surrendering, Djokovic turned inward. Through self-awareness and a deep dive into his bodily needs, he overhauled his diet, his mental conditioning, and subsequently, his tennis game.

The transformation was nothing short of miraculous. Djokovic went on to dominate the tennis world, racking up Grand Slam titles and proving that a strong mind-body connection could dramatically alter your life and career. If Djokovic hadn't paid attention to the messages his body was sending him, if he hadn't altered his mental game, would he have risen to the same heights? Most likely not.

## Mindfulness: The First Step to Intention Setting

Setting intentions starts with being aware—mindful of your current state, your goals, and the path that connects the two. When you lift a dumbbell, is it just an upward and downward motion of your arm, or is it a conscious engagement of your bicep muscle? The difference between the two is mindfulness —being present in the moment, fully engaged in the action at hand.

## Detailed Explanations: The Intention-Action Gap

Ever decided to lose weight, felt incredibly motivated, but found yourself eating a bag of chips a day later? That's the intention-action gap. Good intentions are the starting point, but how do you make them stick? By attaching them to something tangible, something actionable. This is where the 'Mind-Body Contract' comes into play.

## The Mind-Body Contract

It's an agreement between your intentions and your actions. If your intention is to 'lose weight,' translate it into action: 'I will walk 10,000 steps a day' or 'I will replace dessert with fruit four times a week.' It's not wishful thinking; it's a promise to yourself, a contract.

## Daily Tasks and Training Program to Harness Mind-Body Connection

- **Morning Meditation:** Start with 5-10 minutes of mindfulness meditation to set the tone for the day.

- **Intention Journal:** Before you start your workout, jot down what you intend to achieve through it. Are you looking to build endurance, gain strength, or boost your mood?

- **Active Awareness:** During your regular workout, set aside one session per week as your 'Awareness Workout.' During this session, focus solely on your form, your breath, and the muscles you're engaging.

- **Reflection Time:** After your workout, take 5 minutes to reflect on what you've achieved and how it aligns with your bigger fitness goals.

## Actionable Strategies

1. **Create a Mind-Body Vision Board:** A collage of images, quotes, and reminders of your fitness goals can keep your intentions in sight.

2. **Turn Intentions Into Mantras:** Use affirmations to turn your intentions into something memorable, e.g., 'Every step I take brings me closer to my best self.'

3. **Seek Professional Guidance:** Sometimes our own minds can be our worst enemies. Therapists or life coaches can offer valuable perspectives on setting and achieving intentions.

## Food for Thought

- Are your intentions rooted in self-improvement or are they imposed by societal pressures?
- How do your daily actions validate or betray your intentions?

## Summary

1. **The Mind is Your Rudder:** Direct it wisely to sail smoothly toward your fitness goals.

2. **Real-world Proof:** Novak Djokovic's career skyrocketed when he made a conscious effort to align his mind and body.

3. **Mastering Mindfulness:** Being aware of your present actions is the first step toward intentional living.

4. **Closing the Intention-Action Gap:** Your Mind-Body Contract translates vague intentions into tangible actions.

5. **Daily Practices & Actionable Strategies:** Mindfulness meditation, intention journaling, and active awareness during workouts can anchor your mind-body connection.

6. **Questions to Ponder:** Constantly evaluate whether your intentions and actions are aligned with your true self.

Your journey to fitness is not merely a physical one; it's a psychological expedition too. By focusing on the mind-body connection, you equip yourself with the most potent tool available—conscious intention. Much like Novak Djokovic, you have the potential to revolutionize your life. All it takes is a bit of inner alignment and a whole lot of conscious action. Your body is ready; it's time to get your mind on board!

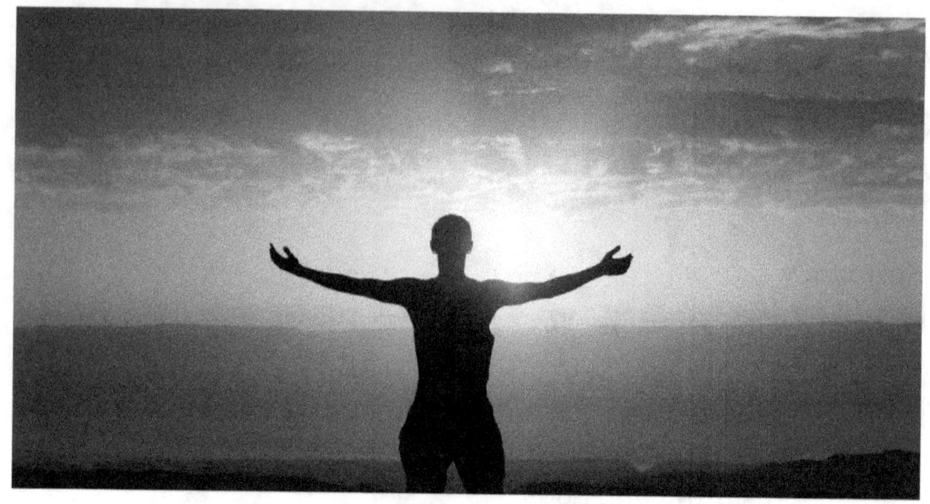

*Chapter 3:*

*The Importance of Goal Setting*

## An Expedition Requires a Map

Imagine you're embarking on a hike through a dense, uncharted forest. You wouldn't dare to set out without a map, a compass, or some form of guidance. The journey to optimum fitness is no different. Goals serve as your roadmap, your North Star, guiding you through the wilderness of challenges, temptations, and setbacks. Without clear goals, you're like a ship sailing aimlessly, subject to the whims of the wind and waves.

## Michael Phelps: The Power of Clear Goals

Who better to exemplify the sheer power of goal setting than Michael Phelps, the most decorated Olympian of all time? But the path to 23 gold medals wasn't strewn with roses; it was riddled with challenges, one of which was Attention Deficit Hyperactivity Disorder (ADHD).

As a child, Phelps had trouble focusing, but his mother

was committed to channeling his energy into something constructive. Cue swimming. Phelps' goal? To master the art of focus through swimming. With this clear objective, he, his mother, and his coaches crafted a meticulous plan, including 6-hour practices six days a week. He even had a goal sheet that he kept in his bedroom, with times he wanted to achieve in various events.

The result? His name became synonymous with excellence in swimming. Every stroke in the pool was a step toward his goals; every lap was a building block for his Olympic dreams. His journey demonstrates that setting a clear, achievable goal can not only guide you but can transform your life.

## SMART Goals: The Gold Standard

You've likely heard of SMART goals: Specific, Measurable, Achievable, Relevant, and Time-bound. This isn't some corporate jargon; it's a valuable method for goal setting that applies splendidly to your fitness journey.

## Detailed Explanation of SMART Goals

1. **Specific:** Instead of saying, "I want to get fit," say, "I want to lose 10 pounds and run a 5K in under 30 minutes."

2. **Measurable:** How will you track your progress? Perhaps through weekly weigh-ins or time trials.

3. **Achievable:** Is your goal realistic given your current fitness level, time commitments, and resources?

4. **Relevant:** Does your goal align with your broader lifestyle and long-term ambitions?

5. **Time-bound:** When do you aim to accomplish your goal? Assign a specific date.

## Daily Tasks and Training Program: Goals at a Micro Level

- **Morning Assessment:** Take a few minutes each morning to evaluate your daily objectives. What can you do today to come one step closer to your goal?

- **Activity Tracker:** Wear a fitness tracker to monitor your physical activity. Aim to hit specific targets each day, like 30 minutes of aerobic exercise.

- **Nutritional Goals**: Plan your meals for the day with a specific target in mind—perhaps it's cutting out sugar or ensuring you get 30 grams of protein.

## Actionable Strategies

1. **Visualize Your Goals:** Create a vision board with images that depict your fitness goals. Look at it daily to keep your objectives top-of-mind.

2. **Accountability Partner:** Having someone to share your journey can make all the difference. Regularly update them on your progress, and allow them to do the same.

3. **Celebratory Milestones**: Reward yourself for small victories on your path to your larger goal. Hit your first 5K? Treat yourself to a new pair of running shoes.

## Food for Thought

- Do your goals truly resonate with what you want, or are they influenced by external factors like societal norms or peer pressure?

- Does the fear of not achieving your goals deter you from setting them in the first place?

## Summary

1. **Navigational Tools:** Goals act as your roadmap in the journey of fitness, preventing you from going astray.

2. **The Phelps Phenomenon:** Michael Phelps shows us how meticulous goal-setting can lead to world records and personal transformation.

3. **SMART Goals:** Specificity, measurability, achievability, relevance, and time constraints are the building blocks of effective goals.

4. **Daily Habits & Training Program:** From morning assessments to activity tracking and nutrition planning, everyday actions should align with your overarching goals.

5. **Actionable Strategies:** Visualization, accountability, and small rewards keep you on track and motivated.

Goals are the fuel that propels you forward in your fitness journey. They offer structure to your aspirations and provide a quantitative measure of your progress. By setting SMART goals, breaking them down into daily tasks, employing actionable strategies, and, most importantly, aligning them with your deepest desires, you can achieve more than you ever thought possible.

Remember, a goal without a plan is just a wish. So stop wishing and start planning; your best self awaits, and the path to it is paved with well-set goals.

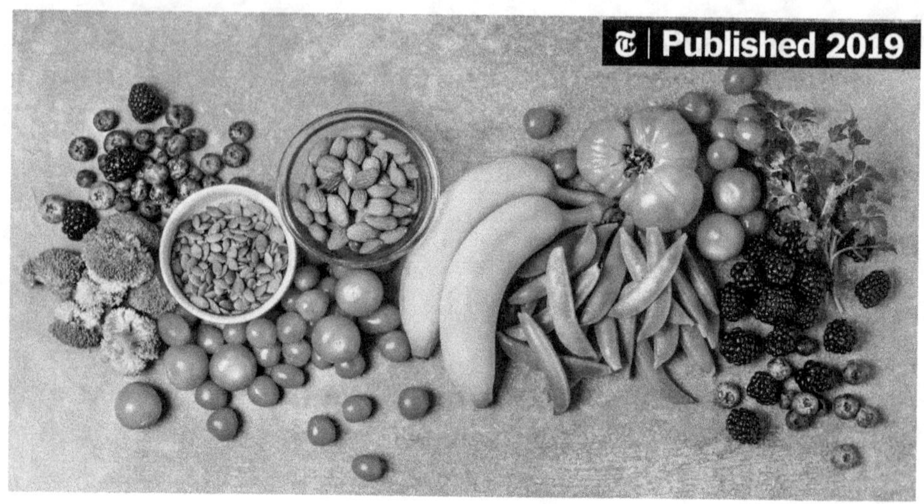


*Chapter 4:*

*Basics of Nutrition*

## The Fuel That Powers You

Would you pour soda into your car's fuel tank and expect it to run efficiently? The answer is obvious: absolutely not. Yet many of us overlook the vital role that nutrition plays in our fitness journey. While workouts sculpt your physique and boost your stamina, it's nutrition that fuels these activities and aids recovery. Simply put, if exercise is the engine, then nutrition is the fuel.

## The Astonishing Transformation of Hugh Jackman

Think of the last time you saw Hugh Jackman play Wolverine in the X-Men series. The sheer bulk and raw muscle he displayed didn't just happen in the gym; they were sculpted in the kitchen as well. Jackman followed a regimented diet that was as rigorous as his workout plan. High in protein, low in unnecessary fats and carbs—his diet was meticulously calculated to help him gain muscle mass and minimize body fat. Even more impressively, Jackman incorporated 'Intermittent Fasting,' only eating within an 8-hour window and fasting for the remaining 16 hours of the day. The result? A physique that's become iconic in Hollywood.

If an actor in his late 40s could transform himself so drastically through nutrition, imagine what thoughtful eating could do for you.

## Macronutrients and Micronutrients: The Building Blocks

### Detailed Explanation

### Macronutrients:

1. **Protein**: Essential for muscle repair and growth. Examples include lean meat, fish, and plant-based proteins like legumes and nuts.

2. **Carbohydrates:** Your body's primary source of energy. Think whole grains, fruits, and vegetables.

3. **Fats:** Necessary for hormone production and nutrient absorption. Opt for healthy fats like those in avocados, olive oil, and fatty fish.

### Micronutrients:

1. **Vitamins:** Necessary for various bodily functions including immune response (Vitamin C), vision (Vitamin A), and bone health (Vitamin D).

2. **Minerals:** Important for nerve function (sodium, potassium), bone health (calcium), and oxygen transport (iron).

## Daily Tasks and Training Program: Nutrition Edition

- **Morning Ritual:** Start your day with a glass of water and a balanced meal that includes all three macronutrients.

- **Meal Prep:** Take time on weekends to prepare your meals for the week. This can be as simple as chopping veggies or as complex as making full meals.

- **Nutrient Timing:** If possible, try to consume protein within a 30-minute window after your workout for optimal muscle recovery.

## Actionable Strategies

1. **Ditch the Junk:** Eliminate or significantly reduce processed foods high in sugar, salt, and unhealthy fats from your diet.

2. **Read Labels**: Before purchasing any packaged food, read the nutrition label. Look for hidden sugars, high sodium levels, and unhealthy fats.

3. **Portion Control:** Use measuring cups or a food scale to get an accurate idea of serving sizes.

## Food for Thought

- How much does convenience factor into your current food choices, and what can you do to make nutritious options more accessible?

- Can you identify any emotional triggers that lead to unhealthy eating? How can you manage these triggers differently?

## Summary

1. **Importance of Nutrition**: Just like a car needs quality fuel to run efficiently, your body requires proper

nutrition to function at its best.

2. **Celebrity Transformation:** Hugh Jackman's physique for the role of Wolverine serves as a testament to the power of a well-planned diet.

3. **Macros & Micros:** Understanding the basic building blocks of nutrition—proteins, carbohydrates, fats, vitamins, and minerals—can help you make informed choices.

4. **Daily Tasks**: From morning rituals to meal prepping and nutrient timing, incorporating these tasks into your routine can make a significant difference in your nutritional habits.

5. **Actionable Strategies**: Eliminating junk, reading food labels, and controlling portions can set you on the right path to better nutrition.

In the grand tapestry of fitness, nutrition forms the threads that hold everything together. Understanding the basics of nutrition can not only expedite your journey to optimal health but can also improve the quality of your life in ways you've never imagined. Whether it's the Herculean physique of Hugh Jackman or the everyday individual aiming for better health, the transformation starts on your plate. So the next time you find yourself mindlessly munching on a bag of chips, remember: you have the power to choose better fuel. Your future self will thank you.

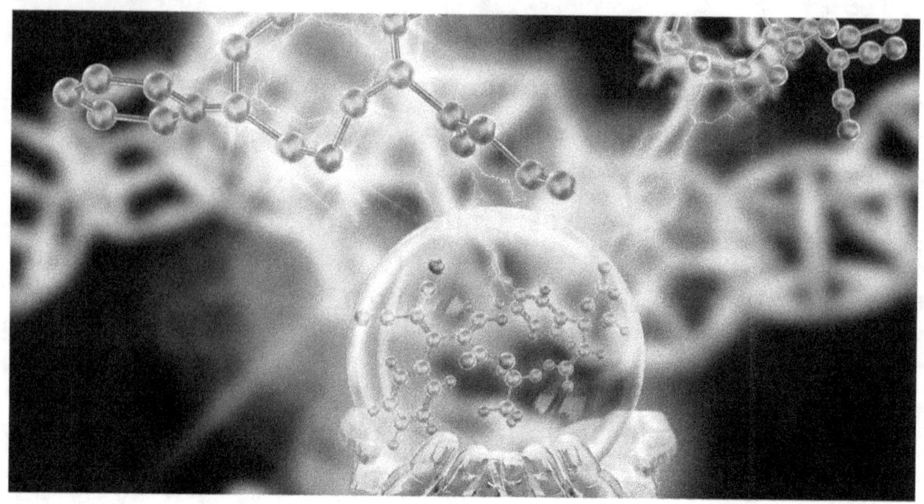

*Chapter 5:*

*The Science of Metabolism*

## The Body's Powerhouse

Imagine if your body were a factory. A complex network of machines, conveyor belts, and control rooms all buzzing with activity, working around the clock to produce energy. This incredible factory is your metabolism, the biochemical process responsible for converting nutrients into the energy that powers everything you do, from exercising to simply breathing.

The Rock's Caloric Symphony: Dwayne Johnson's Masterful Metabolism

Let's talk about Dwayne "The Rock" Johnson, the WWE wrestler turned Hollywood superstar. Have you ever wondered how he maintains that gargantuan physique while working on grueling film sets? The answer lies in his expert manipulation of metabolism. To sustain his muscle mass, Johnson consumes an astounding 5,000-plus calories a day spread over seven meals. But this isn't just a free-for-all buffet; it's a carefully calculated intake of proteins, fats, and carbohydrates designed to optimize his metabolic rate. Even more fascinating is his "cheat day," where he devours mountains of sushi or stacks of pancakes, keeping his metabolism guessing and fired up.

In essence, The Rock has turned his metabolism into a finely-tuned instrument, capable of converting massive amounts of food into muscle and energy with minimal fat storage. But you don't have to be a movie star to master your metabolism; with the right understanding and strategy, anyone can do it.

## The Three Components of Metabolism

### Detailed Explanation

1. **Basal Metabolic Rate (BMR):** This is the amount of energy, in calories, your body requires at rest to maintain basic functions like breathing, circulating blood, and regulating body temperature.

2. **Physical Activity Level (PAL):** The calories you burn through physical exercise.

3. **Thermic Effect of Food (TEF):** The energy required to digest, absorb, and distribute the nutrients in the food you consume.

## Daily Tasks and Training Program: Stoke Your Metabolic Fire

- **Consistent Exercise:** Aim for at least 30 minutes of moderate exercise most days of the week to increase your PAL.

- **Protein-Focused Meals:** Consuming more protein can boost your TEF, as it takes more energy to digest compared to fats and carbs.

- **Hydration:** Drinking cold water can temporarily spike your BMR, helping you burn more calories.

## Actionable Strategies

1. **Eat More, Not Less:** Skipping meals can decrease your BMR, making it harder to lose weight. Aim for smaller, more frequent meals.

2. **High-Intensity Interval Training (HIIT):** This type of exercise can rev up your metabolism for hours after the workout is done.

3. **Get Your Zzz's:** Lack of sleep can mess with the hormones that regulate your metabolism, so aim for at least 7-8 hours a night.

## Food for Thought

- Have you ever tried extreme calorie restriction to lose weight? How did that affect your energy levels and weight loss journey?

- What are some ways you can incorporate more physical activity into your daily routine to boost your metabolism?

## Summary

1. **The Metabolic Factory:** Your metabolism is a complex biochemical process that converts nutrients into energy, powering every function in your body.

2. **Celebrity Spotlight:** Dwayne "The Rock" Johnson optimizes his metabolism by eating over 5,000 calories per day, strategically composed to build muscle and provide energy.

3. **Three Components**: Understanding the role of BMR, PAL, and TEF can help you effectively manage your metabolic rate.

4. **Daily Tasks**: Regular exercise, protein-focused meals, and hydration are key tasks that can positively impact your metabolism.

5. **Actionable Strategies:** Eating more frequent, smaller meals, engaging in HIIT, and prioritizing sleep can all contribute to a healthier metabolism.

If you've always wondered why some people can eat like there's no tomorrow and not gain a pound, while others struggle with weight management, know this: metabolism is not a matter of fate but of science and strategy. Whether you're looking to lose weight, gain muscle, or simply lead a healthier life, understanding the science of metabolism can provide invaluable insights into how your body utilizes energy.

In a world obsessed with diet fads and quick fixes, it's empowering to turn to science as your guide. With a deeper understanding of the factors that influence your metabolic rate, you can customize a strategy tailored to your needs, much like Dwayne Johnson has. After all, your body is an amazing, complex machine—doesn't it deserve the best fuel and maintenance possible?

So as you sip that cold water or finish that last sprint, remember: you're not just sweating; you're stoking the furnace of your metabolic factory, each drop of sweat propelling you closer to your health and fitness goals. And that is truly something to be celebrated.

# PART II: EXERCISE FUNDAMENTALS

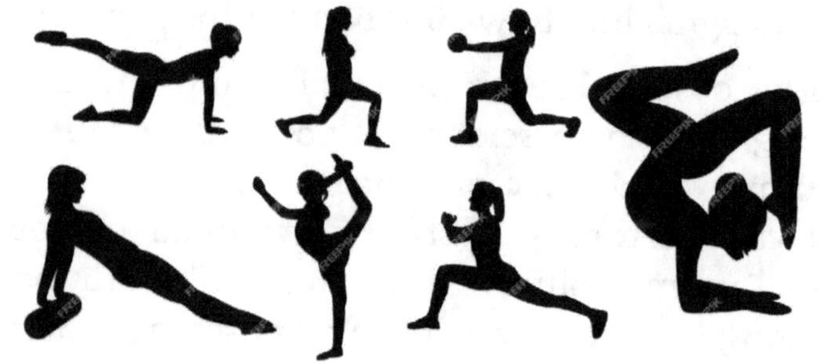

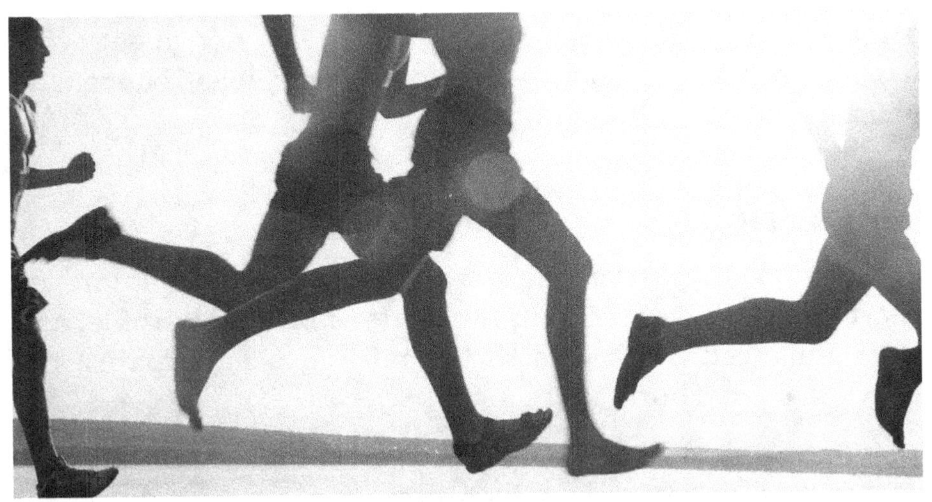

*Chapter 6:*

*Getting Started with Cardio*

## Your Heart, the Unsung Hero

When you think of strength, what comes to mind? Probably bulging biceps or a six-pack abdomen. But what about the incredible strength of your heart, the muscular organ working tirelessly to pump blood through miles of arteries and veins? Cardiovascular exercise—or simply, cardio—is the salute to this unsung hero of your body, and in this chapter, we're diving deep into how to make the most of it.

## From Couch to 5K: The Sarah Reinertsen Story

If you're looking for inspiration, you don't have to look any further than Sarah Reinertsen, an Ironman triathlete. Born with a tissue disease that led to the amputation of her left leg above the knee, she could have easily stayed within her comfort zone. But she chose otherwise. Not only did she embrace cardio, but she also competed and completed an Ironman Triathlon—a feat that includes a 2.4-mile swim, a 112-mile bike ride, and a marathon (26.2 miles). Her message? "It's not about what happens to you. It's about what you do with what happens to you."

## Why Cardio?

Cardiovascular exercise offers a plethora of benefits: improved heart health, increased stamina, better hormonal profile, and even enhanced mood due to the release of endorphins, the body's feel-good hormones.

## Detailed Explanation: Types of Cardio

1. **Steady-State Cardio:** This is your traditional, moderate-intensity cardio. Think a 30-minute jog or a long bike ride.

2. **High-Intensity Interval Training (HIIT):** Short bursts of extreme intensity followed by rest or low-intensity periods. For example, 30 seconds of sprinting followed by 30 seconds of walking.

3. **Circuit Training:** A series of exercises performed one after the other with little to no rest in between.

## Daily Tasks and Training Program

- **Morning Jog:** Start your day with a 20-30 minute jog at a moderate pace.

- **Lunchtime Walk:** A 10-minute walk post-lunch can not only aid digestion but also contribute to your daily cardio.

- **Evening HIIT:** Twice a week, engage in a 20-minute HIIT session to ramp up fat loss and improve cardiovascular health.

## Actionable Strategies

1. **Heart Rate Monitoring:** Wearing a heart rate monitor can help you ensure you're exercising at the right intensity for maximum benefits.

2. **Change It Up:** The body adapts quickly. Switch between different types of cardio to keep your body guessing.

3. **Consult a Professional:** Especially if you're new to cardio or have any health issues, consulting a physician or a certified trainer is advisable.

## Food for Thought

- How can you integrate cardio seamlessly into your day? Could you possibly bike to work, or take the stairs instead of the elevator?

- Sarah Reinertsen turned a seeming limitation into a springboard for greatness. What limitations could you turn into stepping stones?

## Summary

1. **Importance of Cardio:** Cardiovascular health is crucial for overall well-being and life longevity.

2. **Real-life Hero:** Sarah Reinertsen defied all odds and became an Ironman triathlete, proving that limitations can be stepping stones.

3. **Types of Cardio:** From steady-state to HIIT and circuit training, understanding the various types of cardio can guide you to make an informed choice.

4. **Daily Tasks:** Incorporating cardio into your daily routine can be as easy as morning jogs, lunchtime walks, or evening HIIT sessions.

5. **Actionable Strategies:** Monitoring your heart rate, switching your routine, and consulting professionals can optimize your cardio regimen.

Starting a cardio regimen can feel daunting, but remember, every heart-pounding moment is a love letter to your health and well-being. Whether you're an aspiring Ironman like Sarah Reinertsen or just someone looking to elevate your fitness game, there's a type of cardio that's perfect for you.

Sarah Reinertsen's story teaches us that the most formidable barriers often reside in our minds. Break those barriers, and the path is as clear as the road ahead during an early morning jog. She didn't let her physical condition define her; instead, she redefined what's possible through sheer will, training, and an unbreakable spirit. You have that same spirit within you, and cardio can be the key to unlocking it.

So go ahead, lace up those running shoes and hit the pavement. Your heart will thank you, your body will transform, and your spirit will soar. Because remember, in the grand narrative of your life, cardio isn't just a chapter; it's a recurring theme that makes the entire story better.

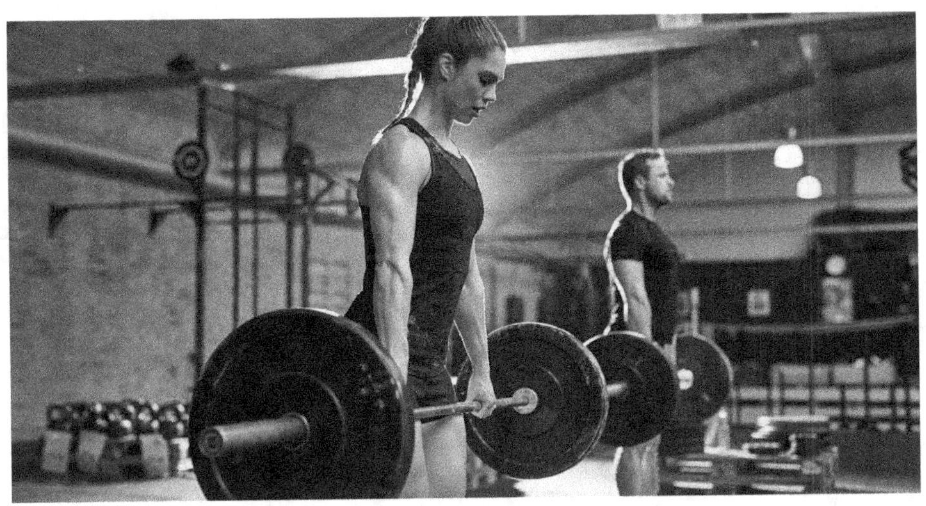

## Chapter 7:

## Strength Training 101

**Unraveling the Muscle Mystery**

Why is strength training often met with such trepidation? For many, the term conjures images of bulky bodybuilders or gym rats who spend all day lifting heavy weights. But the truth is, strength training isn't just about "getting ripped" or bench pressing a small car. It's about improving your quality of life, from carrying groceries with ease to boosting your metabolism and even enhancing your mental well-being.

**The Legend of Schwarzenegger: A Transformation Journey**

Arnold Schwarzenegger's story reads like a modern-day odyssey. From a young Austrian boy with a dream to Mr. Olympia, and from Hollywood icon to the Governor of California, Arnold's life showcases what strength training can lead to. Sure, his physique is legendary, but his approach to strength training transcended mere aesthetics. He viewed each workout as a step towards mastery, not just of his body, but of his life's goals. Schwarzenegger often says, "The resistance that you fight physically in the gym and the resistance that you fight in life can only build a strong character."

## The Myriad Benefits of Strength Training

Strength training benefits extend well beyond muscle development. The activity is known to improve bone density, increase metabolic rate, improve cognitive function, and even aid in the prevention of chronic diseases like diabetes and heart disease.

## Detailed Explanation: Types of Strength Training

1. **Resistance Machines:** These are specialized machines that target specific muscle groups, like the leg press machine for your quads.

2. **Free Weights:** This category includes dumbbells, barbells, and kettlebells. Free weights engage more stabilizer muscles, making the workout more holistic.

3. **Bodyweight Exercises:** Think push-ups, pull-ups, and squats. Your own body provides the resistance.

## Daily Tasks and Training Program

## For Beginners: 3-day Split

- **Day 1: Upper Body**
  - Bench Press: 3 sets of 10 reps
  - Dumbbell Rows: 3 sets of 10 reps
  - Bicep Curls: 3 sets of 12 reps
- **Day 2: Lower Body**
  - Squats: 3 sets of 10 reps

- Leg Curls: 3 sets of 12 reps
- Calf Raises: 3 sets of 15 reps
- **Day 3: Core and Cardio**
  - Planks: 3 sets of 30 seconds
  - Russian Twists: 3 sets of 16 reps
  - 20 minutes of steady-state cardio

## Actionable Strategies

1. **Consistency Over Intensity:** As a beginner, focus more on consistency rather than lifting heavy weights.

2. **Rest and Recovery:** Always have at least one rest day between strength-training workouts to allow for muscle recovery.

3. **Nutrition Matters:** Protein aids in muscle recovery and growth. Aim for at least 1.6 to 2.2 grams of protein per kilogram of body weight.

## Food for Thought

- How do you perceive strength training? Is it an intimidating concept, or do you see it as an empowering way to gain control over your body?

- Schwarzenegger saw resistance as an opportunity to build character. What are the resistances you are facing today, and how can you use them to your advantage?

## Summary

1. **Demystifying Strength:** Strength training isn't just for bodybuilders; it's for anyone who wishes to improve their quality of life.

2. **The Schwarzenegger Way:** Arnold's journey

exemplifies how strength training can be a stepping stone to achieving greater things in life.

3. **Types of Training:** Whether you choose resistance machines, free weights, or bodyweight exercises, the key is to find what suits you best.

4. **Daily Program:** A beginner-friendly 3-day split can set you on the path to a stronger, healthier you.

5. **Actionable Steps:** Prioritize consistency, allow for rest days, and don't forget the importance of nutrition in your strength training journey.

If you have doubts about the relevance of strength training in your life, remember Arnold Schwarzenegger's philosophy. Strength training for him wasn't just a means to an end; it was a transformative experience that fed into all aspects of his life. And there's no reason it can't be the same for you.

The weights in the gym are much like the challenges in life—both require your focus, energy, and sustained effort to overcome. Each lift, each grunt, and each drop of sweat is a small but definitive step towards a stronger, more resilient you. Strength training, therefore, becomes not just a physical endeavor but a holistic experience that tunes your body, sharpens your mind, and builds your character.

So don your workout gear and grip that barbell, for you're not just lifting metal; you're lifting your life to a whole new plane. As you push against the resistance, you'll find that it's not just your muscles that grow, but your self-esteem, your confidence, and your outlook towards life.

Strength training is not a chapter in your life; it's a lifestyle. Commit to it, and you'll discover that the heaviest weights you lift are not the dumbbells or the barbells, but your own limitations.

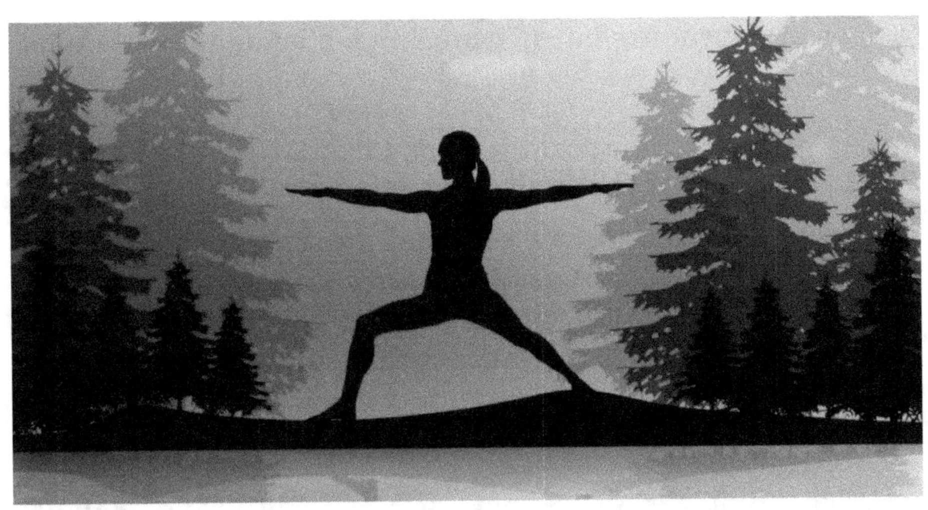

*Chapter 8:*

*Flexibility and Balance*

## The Symphony of Movement

Flexibility and balance might not have the flash of a high-speed treadmill session or the grunt of a heavy lifting set, but they are the unsung heroes that keep the whole operation running smoothly. Just as a world-class symphony isn't just about the soloists but also about the harmonious interplay of all instruments, a well-rounded fitness routine isn't complete without flexibility and balance training.

## Stretching Beyond Limits: The Story of Misty Copeland

Misty Copeland, the first African American female principal dancer with the prestigious American Ballet Theatre, is a paragon of both flexibility and balance. But her path to stardom was fraught with challenges, including a late start in ballet training at the age of 13 and a multitude of doubters who felt her body wasn't right for ballet. Her incredible flexibility and balance were not just physical attributes but also metaphors for her life—bending but not breaking, staying poised amidst pressure.

## The Crucial Role of Flexibility and Balance

Flexibility and balance are essential for daily activities, from tying your shoelaces to reaching for a can on the top shelf. They help in injury prevention, improve posture, and enhance physical performance. Flexibility helps with range of motion, while balance keeps you stable and coordinated.

## Detailed Explanation: Types of Flexibility and Balance Exercises

1. **Static Stretching:** Long, extended stretches that are held for at least 30 seconds.

2. **Dynamic Stretching:** Fluid movements where joints and muscles go through a full range of motion, like leg swings or arm circles.

3. **Core Exercises:** Exercises like planks and Pilates movements help in building a stable core, which aids in balance.

4. **Yoga and Tai Chi:** These ancient practices combine flexibility, balance, and mindfulness.

## Daily Tasks and Training Program

### For All Levels: A 7-Day Program

- **Day 1: Yoga Flow**
  - Sun Salutations: 3 rounds
  - Warrior Poses: 3 sets on each side
- **Day 2: Core and Stretch**
  - Plank: Hold for 30-60 seconds

- Hamstring Stretch: 3 sets of 30 seconds
- **Day 3: Dynamic Stretching**
    - Leg Swings: 3 sets of 10 reps each leg
    - Arm Circles: 3 sets of 10 reps
- **Day 4-7: Repeat Days 1-3, adding one more round or set to each exercise.**

## Actionable Strategies

1. **Consistent Practice:** Just like strength training or cardio, flexibility and balance require consistent practice.
2. **Proper Form:** It's better to do a smaller range of motion correctly than a larger one incorrectly. Quality over quantity.
3. **Active Rest Days:** Incorporate flexibility and balance exercises into your rest days.

## Food for Thought

- Misty Copeland turned her flexibility and balance into an art form. What can you achieve by incorporating these aspects into your fitness routine?
- Do you view flexibility and balance as supplementary to your main exercise routine, or could they be the focus?

## Summary

1. **In the Orchestra of Fitness:** Flexibility and balance might not be the soloists, but they're instrumental in keeping the symphony harmonious.
2. **Misty Copeland:** Her life story exemplifies how flexibility and balance can be both a physical attribute

and a life skill.

3. **Types of Exercises:** From stretching to core exercises to Yoga and Tai Chi, there are numerous ways to improve your flexibility and balance.

4. **Daily Program:** A 7-day rotation can keep things fresh and engaging while ensuring that you're consistently improving.

5. **Actionable Strategies:** Consistency, proper form, and making flexibility and balance part of your rest days can go a long way.

Flexibility and balance are more than just attributes; they are philosophies. Misty Copeland didn't just use her physical flexibility to achieve challenging ballet positions; she used her mental flexibility to adapt to challenges and silence doubters. She didn't just use her balance to perform complex dance movements; she used it to keep her life in equilibrium despite the odds against her.

Incorporating flexibility and balance into your life isn't just about preventing injuries or improving your athletic performance; it's about creating a lifestyle that is adaptable, resilient, and poised. It's about learning to bend so you won't break and gaining the balance to move gracefully through life's challenges.

This might require a shift in focus, placing what was once considered peripheral to the center stage. But remember, in a symphony, every instrument, no matter how small, adds depth and richness to the overall sound. In the same way, every aspect of your fitness regimen, including flexibility and balance, contributes to a healthier, stronger, and more harmonious you.

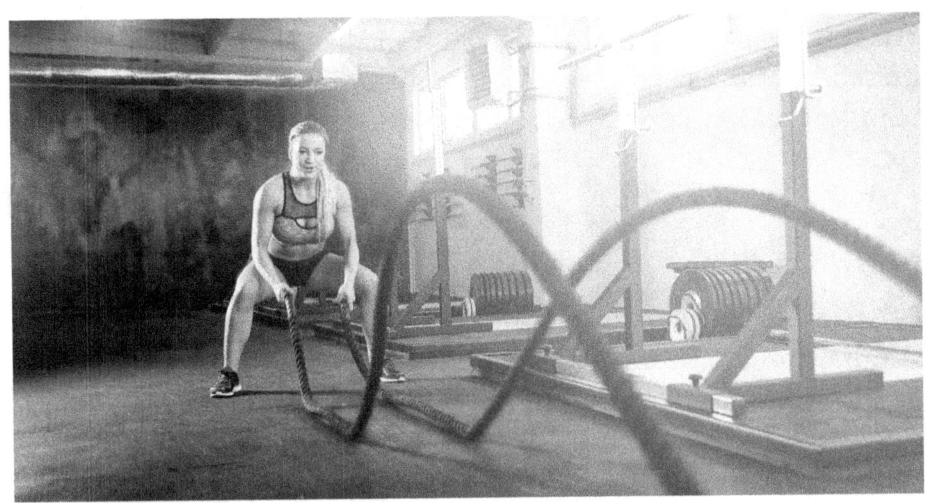

*Chapter 9:*

*Functional Training:*
*Exercise for Daily Life*

## Exercise Beyond Aesthetics

The term "functional training" has become a buzzword in the fitness industry, but its core idea is simple: training your body to be capable and strong in real-world situations. It isn't just about sculpted abs or bulging biceps; it's about enhancing the quality of your everyday life. Imagine lifting your kids without straining your back, carrying groceries with ease, or even having the strength and flexibility to avoid common injuries.

## Real-Life Inspiration: Serena Williams

If you're looking for someone who epitomizes functional strength, look no further than tennis legend Serena Williams. Her training doesn't just involve hitting tennis balls; it includes lifting, plyometrics, and a wide range of functional exercises designed to improve her game and keep her body in top form for daily life. Serena's powerful serves and astonishing agility are the result of training that emphasizes functionality—her incredible fitness translates to more than just winning Grand Slams; it makes her a dynamic and powerful human being in all spheres of life.

## Functional Fitness Defined

Functional training targets multiple muscle groups and joints, simulating common movements you might do at home, work, or in sports. It engages your core, challenges your balance, and requires coordination. Unlike traditional weightlifting, where each muscle might be isolated and worked separately, functional training often involves complex, multi-joint and multi-muscle movements.

## Detailed Explanations

1. **Compound Movements**: Exercises like squats, deadlifts, and lunges are great examples. They work multiple joints and muscles and are fundamental to actions like sitting, standing, and lifting.

2. **Core Stability**: Any movement that requires you to stabilize your spine and pelvis falls under functional training. Planks, bird-dogs, and Russian twists are examples.

3. **Balance and Agility**: Exercises like single-leg stands, ladder drills, and plyometric jumps improve your body's ability to control and stabilize its movements.

## Daily Tasks and Training Program

## Two-Week Functional Training Program

- **Week 1:**

- **Day 1: Lower Body & Core**
  - Squats: 3 sets of 12 reps
  - Planks: 3 sets of 30 seconds
- **Day 2: Upper Body & Balance**
  - Push-ups: 3 sets of 10 reps
  - Single-leg stands: 3 sets of 15 seconds per leg
- **Day 3: Cardio & Agility**
  - Ladder drills: 3 sets
  - 20-minute brisk walk
- **Week 2:**
  - **Day 1: Lower Body & Core**
    - Lunges: 3 sets of 10 reps per leg
    - Russian Twists: 3 sets of 15 reps
  - **Day 2: Upper Body & Balance**
    - Pull-ups or Assisted Pull-ups: 3 sets of 8 reps
    - Bosu ball squats: 3 sets of 12 reps
  - **Day 3: Cardio & Agility**
    - Box Jumps: 3 sets of 10 jumps
    - 20-minute jog

## Actionable Strategies

1. **Incorporate Everyday Movements**: Use exercises that mimic daily activities.

2. **Progressive Overload**: As you get comfortable, add more resistance or complexity to your exercises.

3. **Mix It Up**: Include a variety of exercises to cover all aspects of functional fitness.

## Food for Thought

- How can your fitness routine better prepare you for the movements and activities you encounter in daily life?
- Consider the long-term benefits of functional training. It's not just about immediate gains; it's about life-long abilities and freedoms.

## Summary

1. **Functional Training is a Lifestyle**: It isn't just a set of exercises; it's a mindset geared towards long-term well-being.

2. **Serena Williams as a Model**: Her functional training keeps her not only competitive in tennis but also capable and dynamic in everyday life.

3. **Components of Functional Training**: Compound movements, core stability, and balance and agility are key pillars.

4. **Two-Week Program**: A simple program to introduce you to functional training, covering a variety of movements and muscle groups.

5. **Actionable Steps**: Practical tips to make your training effective and aligned with your daily activities.

Functional training is, in many ways, a return to the roots of physical activity—a far cry from the compartmentalized exercises that occupy many modern gyms. It's about whole-body wellness, preparing you for the complexities of daily life just like Serena Williams prepares for the challenges on the tennis court.

By focusing on functional training, you are not only sculpting your body for today but also preparing it for the future. You're ensuring that you can play with your grandchildren, travel the world, or continue engaging in your favorite activities for years to come. Functional fitness isn't just about the here and now; it's a lifelong investment.

You'll find that as you integrate functional exercises into your routine, not only will your gym performance improve, but the world outside will become a more manageable, less intimidating place. Because at the end of the day, what is fitness if not the ability to navigate the world with strength, ease, and joy?

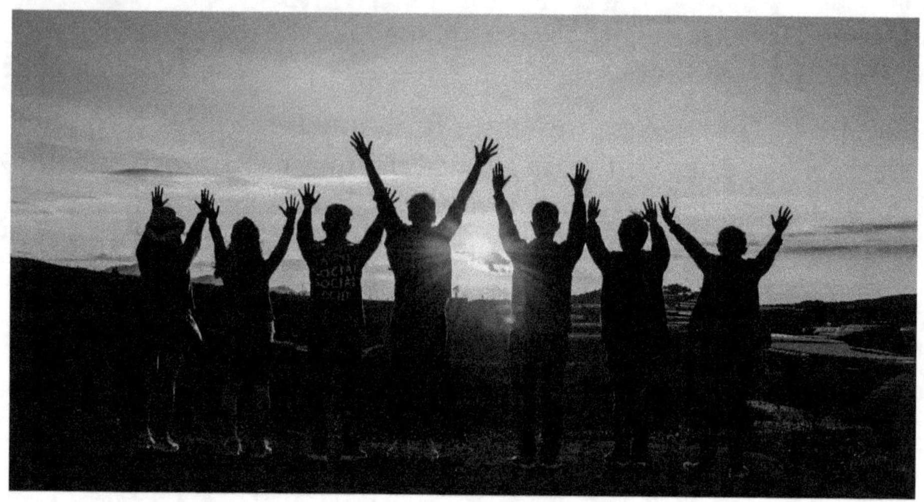

## Chapter 10:

## Workout Plans for Every Lifestyle

### An Introduction to Lifestyle-Focused Fitness

How many times have you heard the phrase, "I don't have time to work out"? In our hectic lives, it's easy to dismiss exercise as a luxury reserved for those with endless hours to spend in the gym. But the truth is, fitness is for everyone, regardless of how busy or relaxed your schedule may be. The key lies in customizing your workout plans to fit seamlessly into your existing lifestyle.

### A Tale of Two Lives: The Rock and Warren Buffett

When you think of Dwayne "The Rock" Johnson, the first image that comes to mind is probably his larger-than-life physique. He often shares snippets of his 4 a.m. workouts, which are intensive and demanding. For The Rock, physical fitness is a non-negotiable part of his day. Contrast this with Warren Buffett, one of the world's richest men, who at 90+ years of age, maintains a different type of routine. While Buffett doesn't pump iron like

Johnson, he keeps his mind sharp and credits his long walks and moderate diet for his physical well-being.

What do these two immensely successful people teach us? That there is no one-size-fits-all when it comes to fitness. Whether you're a CEO, a parent juggling multiple responsibilities, or a college student on a budget, there's a workout plan tailored for your lifestyle.

**Detailed Explanations: The Plans**

*The Busy Bee Plan*

**Duration**: 20-30 minutes

**Frequency**: 3 times a week

**Components**: High-Intensity Interval Training (HIIT), body-weight exercises.

*Sample Workout:*

1. Warm-up (5 minutes)
2. Push-ups (30 seconds)
3. Jump squats (30 seconds)
4. Plank (30 seconds)
5. Burpees (30 seconds)
6. Cool down and stretch (5 minutes)

*The Work-from-Home Warrior Plan*

**Duration**: 45 minutes

**Frequency**: 5 times a week

**Components**: Yoga, Pilates, strength training.

*Sample Workout:*

1. Warm-up (10 minutes of light yoga)
2. Pilates leg series (10 minutes)
3. Dumbbell curls (3 sets of 10)
4. Plank variations (5 minutes)
5. Cool down and stretch (10 minutes)

### *The Retiree Rejuvenator Plan*

**Duration**: 1 hour

**Frequency**: 3-4 times a week

**Components**: Walking, light strength training, flexibility exercises.

*Sample Workout:*

1. Walk (20 minutes)
2. Seated leg lifts (3 sets of 10)
3. Arm circles (3 sets of 10)
4. Gentle yoga stretches (20 minutes)

### Daily Tasks and Actionable Strategies

1. **Identify Your Type**: Before picking a workout plan,

identify what your day looks like. Are you seated for extended periods, or are you always on the move?

2. **Make a Calendar**: Designate specific times in your week for your workout. Make an appointment with yourself.

3. **Incorporate Fitness Snacks**: For the extremely busy, try 5-minute fitness snacks: quick bouts of exercise like push-ups or a brisk walk, sprinkled throughout the day.

## Food for Thought

- Do you find yourself making excuses for not working out due to your lifestyle? If yes, what's stopping you from modifying your workout plan to fit your schedule?

- Exercise doesn't have to be a full-hour commitment. Even 10-15 minutes can make a significant difference. How can you utilize these short periods effectively?

## Summary

1. **Tailored Workouts**: Whether you're an executive like Warren Buffett or an athlete like The Rock, there's a workout plan tailored for you.

2. **The Plans**: Three adaptable plans for the busy bee, the work-from-home warrior, and the retiree offer choices for every lifestyle.

3. **Actionable Strategies**: Identifying your lifestyle type, making a workout calendar, and using fitness snacks can all help incorporate exercise into your day.

4. **Inclusivity**: Exercise is for everyone. No lifestyle is too busy or too relaxed to benefit from regular physical activity.

5. **Time Management**: Using the time you have effectively can make the difference between a sedentary lifestyle and a healthy one.

So, remember, fitness is not a one-size-fits-all endeavor. It's a lifelong commitment that you adapt and grow into. Whether your days are packed with business meetings or leisure walks, there's always room for fitness. The key is to build a plan that works for you—not one that makes you work for it. If Warren Buffett and The Rock can find a way, so can you. Exercise is not about how much time you have; it's about what you do with the time you've got. So go ahead and seize those moments, because a healthier, stronger you awaits!

# PART III: NUTRITION DEEP DIVE

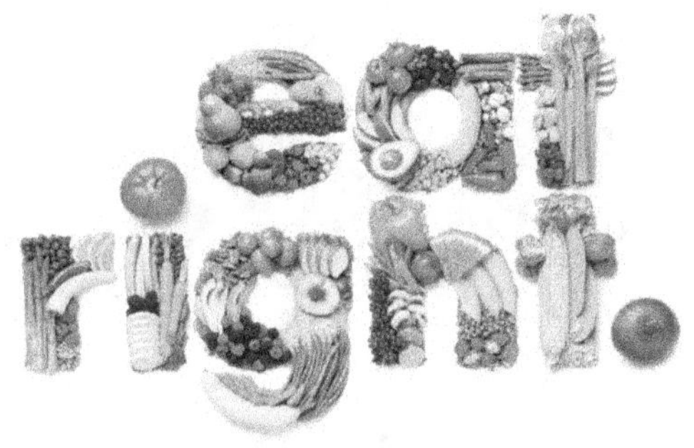

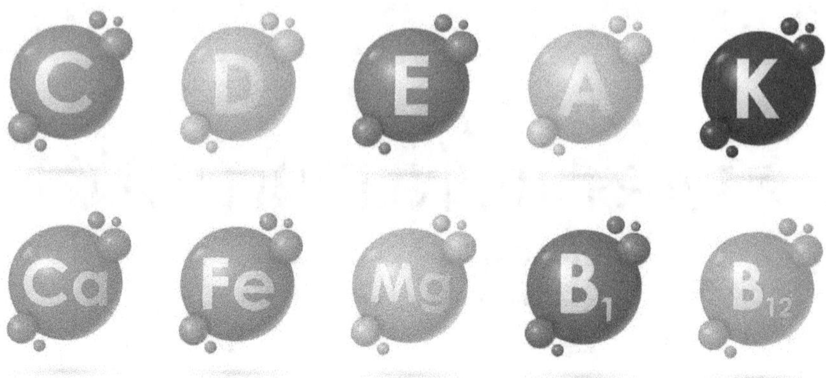

*Chapter 11:*

*Macronutrients Unveiled*

## Decoding the Macronutrient Mystery

When Arnold Schwarzenegger took bodybuilding by storm in the early 1970s, he wasn't just a pioneer in the gym; he was also a pioneer in the kitchen. Arnie was among the first bodybuilders to systematically dial in his protein intake, creating a dietary revolution that echoed through the fitness world. But Schwarzenegger didn't stop at protein; he also understood the critical role of carbohydrates and fats in fueling his workouts and sculpting his legendary physique.

Just as Arnie demystified macronutrients for the Golden Age bodybuilders, this chapter will break down what you need to know about proteins, carbohydrates, and fats, and how they can contribute to your fitness journey.

## What Are Macronutrients?

In simplest terms, macronutrients are the main components of our diet: proteins, carbohydrates, and fats. These are essential for providing energy, building and repairing tissues, and regulating body processes.

## Proteins

**Role**: Primary building blocks for muscle, hormones, enzymes, and more.

**Food Sources**: Meat, fish, dairy, legumes, and plant-based protein sources like tofu.

## Carbohydrates

**Role**: The body's preferred source of energy, especially for quick and explosive movements.

**Food Sources**: Grains, fruits, vegetables, and legumes.

## Fats

**Role**: Energy storage, hormone production, and nutrient absorption.

**Food Sources**: Oils, nuts, seeds, fatty fish, and animal fats.

## Detailed Explanations and Daily Plans

### Protein for Progress

If you're looking to gain muscle, the thumb rule is consuming 1.2 to 2.0 grams of protein per kilogram of body weight.

**Daily Task**: Calculate your body weight in kilograms and multiply by 1.2-2.0 to get your target protein intake.

**Training Program**: If you're weight training, try consuming a protein shake within 30 minutes post-workout for optimal muscle repair.

## Carbohydrates for Energy

In terms of carbs, the amount you need will depend on your level of activity.

**Daily Task**: If you're sedentary, aim for 3-5 grams per kilogram of body weight. For moderate to high-intensity workouts, aim for 5-10 grams per kilogram.

**Training Program**: Try eating a carb-rich meal 2-3 hours before a high-intensity workout.

## Fats for Functionality

Healthy fats are crucial for hormone production, brain function, and overall health.

**Daily Task**: Aim for fats to make up 20-35% of your daily caloric intake.

**Training Program**: Incorporate omega-3 fatty acids, found in fish and flaxseeds, into your diet to help with inflammation and recovery.

## Actionable Strategies

1. **Meal Prepping**: Set aside an hour or two during the weekend to prepare balanced meals for the week.
2. **Track Your Intake**: Use apps like MyFitnessPal to track your macronutrient intake.

3. **Diversify**: Make sure to get your macros from a variety of sources to also ensure you're getting necessary vitamins and minerals.

## Food for Thought

- Are you neglecting one of the three macronutrients? If so, why?
- Can you think of creative ways to combine all three macronutrients into every meal?

## Celebrity Spotlight: Tom Brady

While not a bodybuilder, Tom Brady, the legendary NFL quarterback, places a strong emphasis on his diet, which he credits for his astounding longevity in a physically demanding sport. He adheres to a specific, balanced macronutrient ratio, avoiding foods that cause inflammation. Though controversial, his high-fat, moderate-protein, and low-carb diet has been the subject of much discussion. His strict regimen reiterates the importance of macronutrients in physical performance and longevity.

## Summary

1. **What Are Macros**: Proteins, carbs, and fats are the macronutrients essential for bodily functions and energy.

2. **Detailed Plans**: Proteins for muscle growth, carbs for energy, and fats for hormonal balance. Each has its role, and each requires specific daily tasks and training considerations.

3. **Actionable Strategies**: From meal prepping to tracking your daily intake, there are multiple ways to ensure you're getting the right balance.

4. **The Arnie and Brady Effect**: Whether you're a bodybuilder like Arnold Schwarzenegger or an athlete like Tom Brady, understanding your macronutrients is crucial for optimizing performance and well-being.

5. **Questions for You**: Self-assessment is vital. Regularly check whether you're meeting your macronutrient goals and adjust as necessary.

Understanding your macronutrients is like decoding the blueprint for your body's performance, recovery, and overall health. It's time to follow in the footsteps of fitness and athletic legends by getting your macros right. Your body, and your future self, will thank you.

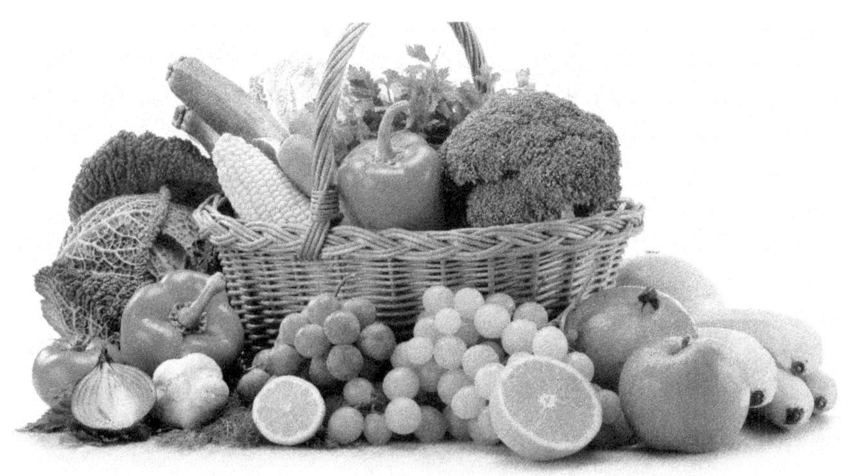

## Chapter 12:

## Vitamins and Minerals

**Introduction: The Unsung Heroes of Nutrition**

We've discussed the heavyweights of the nutrition world: proteins, carbs, and fats. But what about the often-overlooked yet critical aspects of our diet—vitamins and minerals? In the 1960s, Linus Pauling, a Nobel laureate in Chemistry, shook the health world with his advocacy of vitamin C. He claimed that high doses of vitamin C could not only prevent the common cold but could also treat a wide range of diseases, from heart disease to cancer. While the scientific community was skeptical, Pauling brought vitamins front and center in the wellness arena.

In this chapter, we will demystify the role of vitamins and minerals, explain why they are essential for your fitness journey, and share strategies on how to incorporate them into your diet effectively.

***What Are Vitamins and Minerals?***

**Vitamins**

Vitamins are organic compounds that your body needs in small quantities to function correctly. They're critical for energy production, immune function, blood clotting, and more.

## Types of Vitamins:

- Fat-soluble (A, D, E, K)
- Water-soluble (B-complex, C)

## Minerals

Minerals are inorganic elements found in the earth. You need them for bone health, electrolyte balance, and cellular function.

## Types of Minerals:

- Macro-minerals (calcium, magnesium, sodium)
- Trace minerals (iron, zinc, copper)

### *Detailed Explanations and Daily Plans*

### The ABCs of Vitamins

- **Vitamin A**: Necessary for eye health.
  - **Daily Task**: Include orange and dark green vegetables in your diet, like carrots and spinach.
- **B Vitamins**: Essential for energy metabolism.
  - **Daily Task**: Eat whole grains, legumes, and dairy products.
- **Vitamin C**: An antioxidant and immunity booster.
  - **Daily Task**: Eat citrus fruits and berries.

### *Major and Minor Minerals*

- **Calcium**: Important for bone health.
    - **Daily Task**: Include dairy or fortified dairy alternatives in your diet.
- **Iron**: Necessary for oxygen transportation.
    - **Daily Task**: Consume red meat or leafy greens.
- **Zinc**: Essential for immune health.
    - **Daily Task**: Include nuts and seeds in your diet.

## Training Program

- **Pre-Workout**: Ensure you have foods rich in B-vitamins for energy metabolism.
- **Post-Workout**: Calcium-rich foods or shakes can help with bone recovery.

## Actionable Strategies

1. **Supplementation**: If you can't get all the nutrients from food, consider supplements.
2. **Balanced Diet**: Aim for a colorful plate, which often represents a range of vitamins and minerals.
3. **Routine Checks**: Periodic blood tests can determine if you have any deficiencies.

## Celebrity Spotlight: Serena Williams

One of the greatest tennis players of all time, Serena Williams, attributes her longevity and success in part to her meticulous focus on diet and nutrition. She incorporates a balanced amount of vitamins and minerals through both her diet and supplementation. This comprehensive approach helps her recover quickly, maintain high energy levels, and avoid injuries

—critical elements that have contributed to her storied career.

## Food for Thought

- How colorful is your plate? Could it be an indicator of the variety of nutrients you're consuming?
- Is there room for supplementation in your life, or can you get all your vitamins and minerals from food?

## Summary

1. **What are Vitamins and Minerals**: Organic and inorganic compounds necessary for various bodily functions.

2. **Importance**: From bone health to energy metabolism, vitamins and minerals play various roles in your overall health and fitness journey.

3. **Actionable Strategies**: From dietary changes to potential supplementation, various ways ensure you're meeting your vitamin and mineral requirements.

4. **Celeb Factor**: Icons like Serena Williams show that a well-rounded approach to vitamins and minerals can significantly impact performance.

5. **Question Yourself**: Regularly assess your diet and lifestyle to ensure you're not missing out on these essential nutrients.

## Conclusion

Linus Pauling wasn't entirely right about vitamin C's miraculous properties, but he was right about the importance of vitamins and minerals. They may not be as glamorous as macronutrients when we talk about diet and exercise, but they are undeniably essential. By giving these micro but mighty nutrients the attention they deserve, you're setting the stage for a healthier, more vibrant life.

The benefits of adequate vitamin and mineral intake can reverberate through every aspect of your life—from the gym to the office to the comfort of your home. Ignore them at your peril, but embrace them, and you'll find yourself on a well-rounded path to optimal health and fitness.

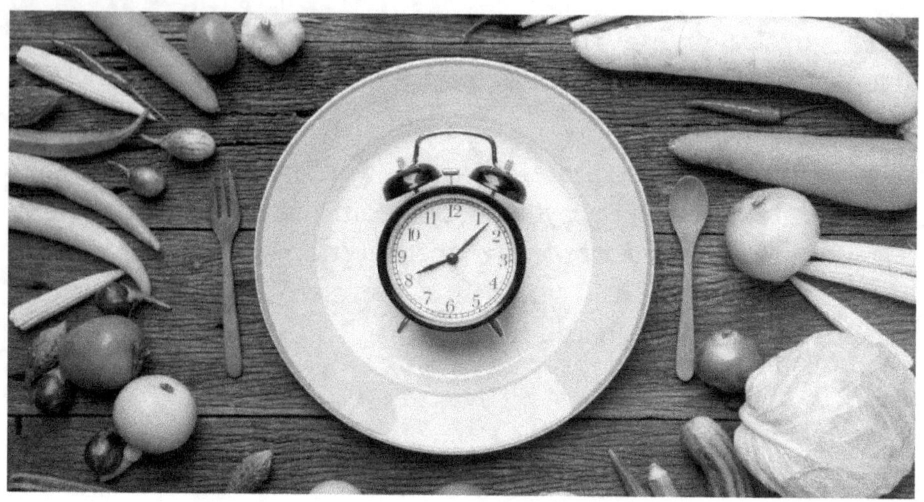

*Chapter 13:*

*Meal Timing and Frequency*

## "What Time Is Chow Time?"

It was 4 a.m., and Dwayne "The Rock" Johnson was already in the gym lifting weights, the clanking of iron echoing through the empty room. By the time most of us hit the snooze button for the first time, he'd already downed his first meal—typically a hefty combo of steak, egg whites, and oatmeal. Now, you may not aspire to be a bodybuilding actor, but The Rock's extreme regimen raises a crucial point: meal timing matters. And it doesn't just matter for elite athletes and Hollywood superstars. It matters for *you.*

## The Science of Meal Timing

Nutrition science has long been preoccupied with *what* we eat. However, emerging research now suggests that *when* we eat can be just as critical. The primary idea behind meal timing is to synchronize your food intake with your body's natural circadian rhythms. You see, your body has internal clocks that regulate everything from sleep to metabolism. When you eat can influence how efficiently your body uses the nutrients.

## When Should You Eat?

Traditional wisdom told us three square meals a day was optimal. However, new perspectives range from intermittent fasting, where one might fast for 16 hours and eat during an 8-hour window, to "grazing," where one might eat smaller meals 5-6 times a day.

## Real-life Anecdote: Emily's Energy Slump

Emily was a busy corporate lawyer, swamped with cases, and fueling her day with vending machine snacks and copious amounts of coffee. She'd skip breakfast, work through lunch, and eat a large dinner. Soon enough, Emily started experiencing energy slumps and weight gain. On a friend's advice, she decided to revamp her eating schedule. She started having a balanced breakfast, a mid-morning snack, a well-portioned lunch, a healthy afternoon snack, and a lighter dinner. Within a few weeks, her energy levels were up, and her scale started tipping in the right direction.

## The Practical Aspect: Daily Tasks and Training Program

**Daily Task 1: Track Your Meals for a Week**: Keep a food diary. When do you feel the most energetic? When do you feel the most sluggish?

**Daily Task 2: Try a New Timing Technique**: For one week, change up your meal timing. If you're a grazer, try three larger meals. If you're a three-meal-a-day person, try smaller meals but increase frequency.

## Training Program:

- **Week 1**: Introduction to meal timing. Maintain your normal diet but adjust the timing of each meal so it aligns with your day's activities.

- **Week 2**: Experiment with intermittent fasting. Choose an 8-hour window that suits your lifestyle and eat within that period.

- **Week 3**: Try the 'six small meals' method. Space out six smaller meals throughout your day.

- **Week 4**: Evaluate. Which meal timing schedule worked best for you? Stick with it for another month and evaluate changes in your energy levels, weight, and overall health.

## Actionable Strategies

1. **Set Alarms**: Use your phone to set mealtime reminders.

2. **Plan Ahead**: Prepare your meals and snacks in advance to align with your meal timing strategy.

3. **Listen to Your Body**: If you find that a particular meal timing method makes you feel lethargic or unwell, switch it up.

## Food for Thought: Circadian Rhythms and Late-Night Snacking

Your body's internal clock doesn't just wake you up or put you to sleep; it also affects your digestion. Studies have shown that late-night eating can lead to weight gain and poor sleep quality. So the next time you reach for that midnight snack, consider whether you're truly hungry or just bored.

## Summary

Meal timing is an underexplored aspect of health and fitness that can make a significant impact on your wellness journey. By synchronizing your meal schedule with your body's natural rhythms, you can optimize nutrient absorption, improve energy levels, and even lose weight. Just like Dwayne "The Rock" Johnson, you too can take control of not just what you eat, but *when* you eat it.

Whether you choose to eat three meals a day, opt for intermittent fasting, or prefer to graze on smaller meals, the key is to be consistent and mindful of how your body reacts to different meal timings. There's no one-size-fits-all answer, but with a bit of experimentation, you can

find the meal timing strategy that works best for you. It's time to sync your internal clock with your mealtime; it's time to make every calorie count.

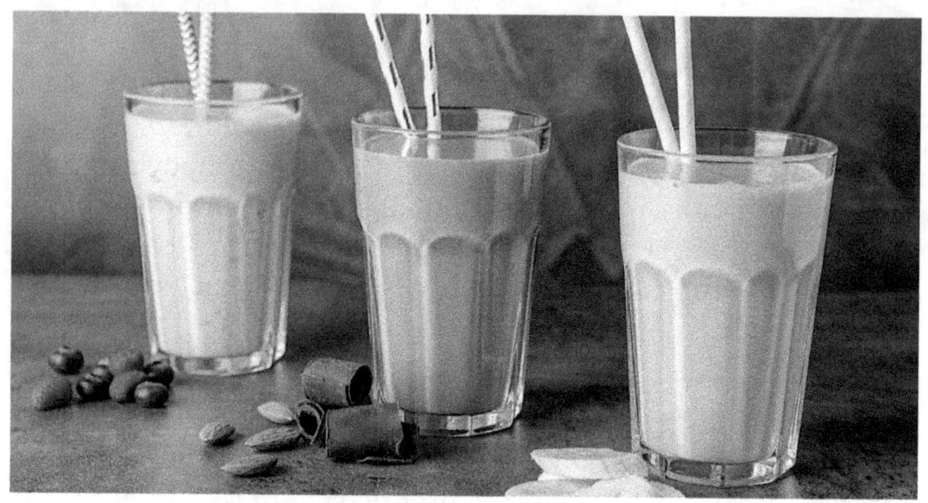

*Chapter 14:*

*Supplements: Do You Need Them?*

**"The Pill That Promises the Moon"**

Imagine for a moment that you're Arnold Schwarzenegger, training for his first Mr. Olympia competition. The room smells of sweat and ambition. Arnold, young but wise, knew something crucial back then: supplements alone don't build champions. Dedication does. He did use supplements, but they were a small piece in a larger puzzle of diet, exercise, and mental preparation.

The market for dietary supplements has exploded into a multi-billion-dollar industry. The aisles of health stores are lined with bottles promising everything from muscle gain to immortal youth. But how many of these supplements do you *actually* need?

**The Science of Supplements**

Before diving into the world of pills, powders, and potions, let's lay down some scientific groundwork. Supplements are meant to *supplement* your diet, not replace real food. For the majority of individuals who eat a balanced diet, supplementation might be unnecessary. But certain groups—athletes, pregnant women, seniors, and those with specific dietary restrictions—may benefit from them.

## Real-life Anecdote: Sam's Iron Misadventure

Meet Sam, an enthusiastic amateur marathon runner. Focused on his protein intake, he neglected other aspects of nutrition. Despite running regularly, Sam felt increasingly fatigued. After some tests, he found out he had an iron deficiency. The doctor recommended an iron supplement along with a balanced diet. Within weeks, Sam's energy levels shot up and his running performance improved.

## What's Worth Your Money?

**1. Protein Powders**: Useful for athletes or fitness enthusiasts who find it hard to meet their protein requirements through food alone.

**2. Omega-3 Fatty Acids**: Essential for heart health and particularly useful for those who don't consume fatty fish regularly.

**3. Multivitamins**: These can be a safety net but are generally not a substitute for a balanced diet.

**4. Creatine**: One of the most researched and supported supplements for muscle gain and performance.

**5. Vitamin D**: Especially useful for those living in areas with limited sun exposure.

**6. Iron and Calcium**: Often recommended for pregnant women or those with specific deficiencies.

## Daily Tasks and Training Program

**Daily Task 1: Audit Your Diet**: Write down everything you eat for three days. Use an app to track the micronutrients you may be missing.

**Daily Task 2: Consult a Professional**: Before starting any new supplement regimen, consult with a healthcare provider.

## Training Program:

- **Week 1**: Introduction to supplements. Start with a basic multivitamin and observe how your body reacts.
- **Week 2**: Add an Omega-3 supplement. Monitor changes in energy and focus.
- **Week 3**: Depending on your fitness goals, add either a protein powder or a specialized supplement like creatine or branched-chain amino acids (BCAAs).
- **Week 4**: Evaluate. Sit down to assess the changes you've noticed since introducing supplements. Are they worth the cost and effort?

## Actionable Strategies

1. **Be Skeptical**: Always question a supplement's promises and read scientific reviews where possible.
2. **Quality Over Quantity**: Choose reputable brands that have been third-party tested for purity.
3. **Start Small**: Introduce one supplement at a time to monitor its effects on your body.

## Food for Thought: The Placebo Effect

In a fascinating study, participants who were given a sugar pill but told it was a performance-enhancing drug showed significant improvements in a physical exercise test. The power of belief is not to be underestimated. While this doesn't mean all supplements are placebos, it suggests that our mindset plays a huge role in our physical performance.

## Summary

In a world that often looks for quick fixes and magic pills, it's important to remember that supplements are just that—supplementary. Arnold Schwarzenegger's success didn't hinge on a protein shake; it was the result of consistent hard work, a well-balanced diet, and strategic supplementation. Before you invest in a monthly supply of the latest, greatest supplement, consider whether your basic nutritional needs are being met through whole foods. If they are not, perhaps it's time to reassess your dietary habits before reaching for a pill bottle.

No supplement can replace the fundamental benefits of a balanced diet, adequate sleep, and regular exercise. However, with the right guidance and for the right reasons, certain supplements can be a valuable addition to your wellness journey. But remember, always consult your healthcare provider for tailored advice.

Whether you decide to venture into the world of supplementation or stick to getting your nutrients from whole foods, remember that there is no shortcut to achieving your health and fitness goals. The real secret lies in your dedication to a balanced lifestyle.

The journey to optimal health is a marathon, not a sprint, and it's your daily habits that will carry you across the finish line. Whether you choose to include supplements on your journey is entirely your decision—but either way, make sure it's a well-informed one.

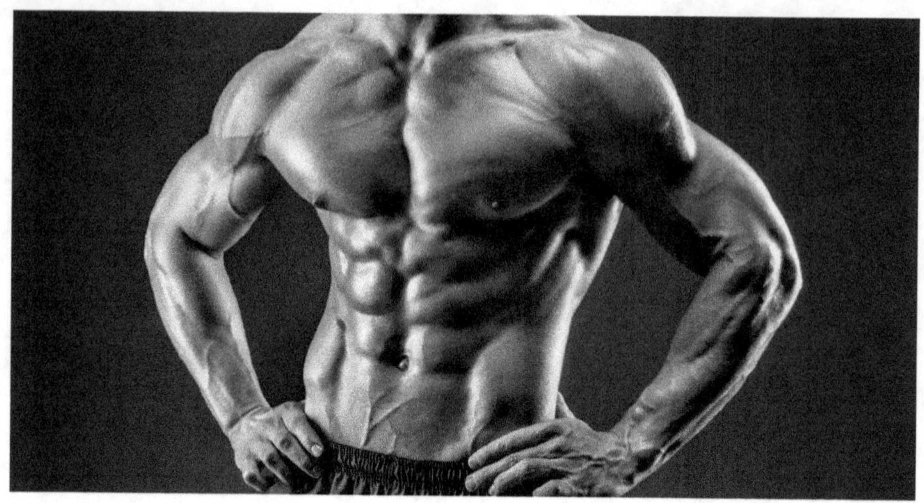

*Chapter 15:*

*Eating for Muscle Gain*

## "When Food Becomes Your Dumbbell"

Imagine stepping into the shoes of Hugh Jackman as he prepared for his iconic role as Wolverine. He had to undergo a jaw-dropping physical transformation, not just through lifting weights but also through eating—lots of eating. Behind those bulging biceps and washboard abs is not just sweat and iron; there's also a meticulously planned, protein-packed diet. If you're after lean muscle, this chapter is your golden ticket.

## The Basic Science: Calories and Macronutrients

When you want to gain muscle, you're essentially asking your body to build new tissue. This requires energy, and energy comes from calories. However, not all calories are created equal. You need a balanced mix of protein for muscle repair, carbohydrates for energy, and fats for overall cellular function.

## Real-life Anecdote: Tim's Protein Epiphany

Tim was a skinny guy who had always struggled to put on muscle. His workouts were intense, but he didn't see the gains he hoped for. One day, his gym buddy suggested tracking his daily protein intake. Tim realized he was only consuming about half the recommended protein for muscle gain. He changed his diet, focusing on lean protein sources, and within weeks, his muscle growth shot up. Tim learned that you can't just train hard; you have to eat right too.

## The Golden Trio for Muscle Gain

**1. Protein**: It's the building block of muscle. Aim for at least 1.6 to 2.2 grams of protein per kilogram of body weight.

**2. Carbohydrates**: They fuel your workouts and help in muscle recovery. Complex carbs like whole grains and starchy vegetables are your best friends.

**3. Fats**: Don't shy away from fats. Your body needs them for hormone production, including hormones like testosterone that are crucial for muscle growth.

## Daily Tasks and Training Program

**Daily Task 1: Track Your Macros**: For one week, use a food tracking app to ensure you're hitting your protein, carb, and fat goals.

**Daily Task 2: Meal Prep**: Dedicate one day a week to meal prepping to ensure you always have muscle-building foods on hand.

## Training Program:

- **Week 1**: Start by calculating your caloric needs for

muscle gain. Add 250-500 calories to your daily caloric maintenance level.

- **Week 2**: Introduce lean protein sources into every meal. Chicken, fish, tofu, and lean beef are good options.

- **Week 3**: Incorporate carb timing. Consume most of your carbs before and after your workouts for optimal muscle recovery.

- **Week 4**: Add healthy fats. Include avocados, nuts, and fatty fish like salmon to meet your daily fat requirements.

## Actionable Strategies

1. **Eat Frequent, Balanced Meals**: Aim for 4-6 meals per day, ensuring each one contains a good balance of protein, carbs, and fats.

2. **Use Protein Shakes Wisely**: If you find it hard to meet your protein requirements through whole foods, consider adding a protein shake as a snack.

3. **Hydrate**: Muscle is about 80% water. Keep hydrated to ensure optimal muscle function and recovery.

## Food for Thought: The 'Dirty Bulk'

The internet is filled with bodybuilders promoting the 'dirty bulk,' where you eat everything in sight to gain mass. While this approach will make the numbers on the scale go up, it's often accompanied by increased body fat and can be detrimental to your long-term health. Remember, quality over quantity.

## Summary

Eating for muscle gain isn't just about piling on the calories;

it's about thoughtful, balanced nutrition. Like Hugh Jackman during his Wolverine prep, gaining muscle is a multi-faceted approach requiring not only disciplined training but also meticulous attention to what you eat.

Your muscle-building journey is as much about what happens in the kitchen as it is about what happens in the gym. Protein is your ally, carbs are your energy source, and fats are the unsung heroes that keep your body functioning smoothly. It's crucial to strike a balance, ensuring that your body has all the raw materials it needs to build muscle efficiently.

Muscle gain isn't rocket science, but it is a science. By understanding the roles of different nutrients and applying the strategies mentioned above, you're setting yourself up for success. But remember, everybody's body responds differently to diet and exercise, so be willing to adjust and adapt your plan as you go along.

Like any well-oiled machine, your body requires the right fuel to function optimally. By giving it what it needs, you'll be well on your way to making noticeable, sustainable muscle gains. So go ahead—eat smart, train hard, and build that muscle you've always dreamed of.

# PART IV: SPECIAL TOPICS

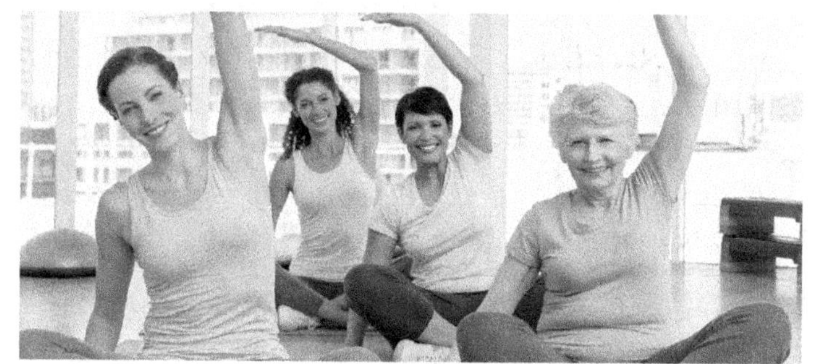

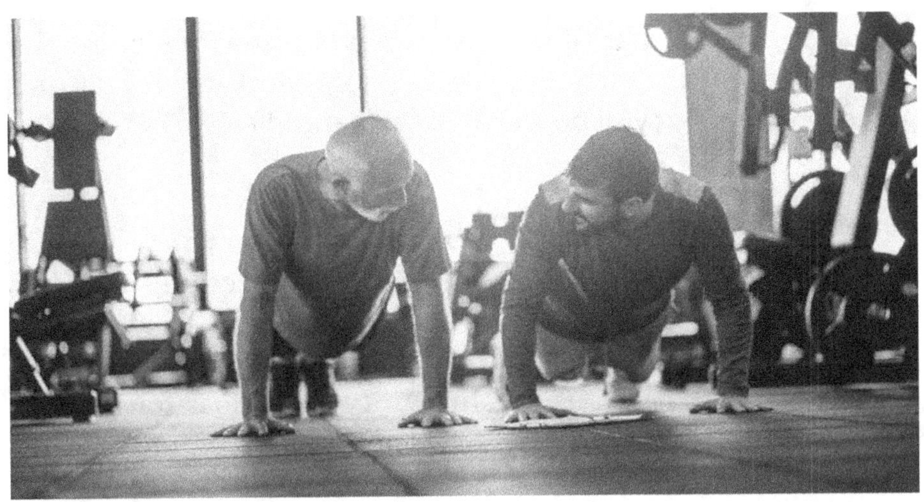

*Chapter 16:*

*Exercise for Seniors*

## "Golden Years, Golden Gains"

Picture this: you're 90-year-old Charles Eugster, standing on the starting line of a 200-meter sprint race. Your competitors are decades younger than you, but the age difference hardly bothers you. Charles, often dubbed the "World's Fittest Nonagenarian," is proof that age is no barrier to physical fitness. With several sprinting records under his belt, he showed that the golden years can indeed be golden.

Let's get one thing straight: You don't have to become an ultra-marathon runner or a weightlifting champion in your later years, but exercise should be a non-negotiable part of your life. As you age, maintaining your physical health becomes increasingly important for overall well-being, mobility, and independence.

## Why Exercise is Critical for Seniors

As we age, muscle mass decreases, bones become fragile, and the metabolism slows down. Exercise can help combat these natural processes, keeping you physically and mentally sharp.

## Real-life Anecdote: Martha's Magical Transformation

Martha was a 72-year-old woman who had accepted that her best years were behind her. She was overweight, had trouble walking, and rarely left her home. On the insistence of her grandchildren, she joined a community yoga class for seniors. Within months, Martha lost weight, her mobility improved, and what's more, her chronic back pain diminished significantly. For Martha, exercise wasn't just a physical savior; it also brought her back into the community.

## Types of Exercises for Seniors

1. **Aerobic Exercise:** Walking, swimming, and cycling are excellent for improving cardiovascular health.
2. **Strength Training:** Light weightlifting or bodyweight exercises help maintain muscle mass.
3. **Flexibility Training:** Yoga and stretching exercises can improve range of motion.
4. **Balance and Coordination:** Exercises like tai chi can prevent falls by improving balance.

## Daily Tasks and Training Program

**Daily Task 1:** Mobility Check: Every morning, perform basic stretches to assess your flexibility and joint health.

**Daily Task 2:** Activity Journal: Maintain an exercise diary to track your progress and set goals.

**Training Program:**

- **Week 1:** Introduction to aerobic exercises. Start with a 10-minute daily walk, gradually increasing the time.
- **Week 2:** Incorporate strength training twice a week. Use resistance bands or light dumbbells for simple exercises like bicep curls and leg raises.
- **Week 3:** Add flexibility exercises. Begin with a 10-minute stretching or yoga routine three times a week.
- **Week 4:** Introduce balance exercises like tai chi or simple balance drills.

## Actionable Strategies

1. **Consult a Physician:** Before beginning any exercise regimen, consult your healthcare provider, especially if you have existing medical conditions.
2. **Start Slow:** Don't jump into an intense routine. Gradually ramp up the activity level to prevent injuries.
3. **Stay Consistent:** Consistency is key, even if it means doing shorter but more frequent exercise sessions.

## Food for Thought: Mindful Movement

As you age, the connection between the mind and body becomes increasingly important. Activities like tai chi and yoga aren't just physical exercises; they also involve mindfulness and focus, which can benefit cognitive function. Exercise is not just about the body; it's also about the mind.

## Summary

Aging is inevitable, but how we age is significantly within our control. Exercise for seniors isn't about becoming the next Charles Eugster; it's about improving the quality of life, maintaining independence, and keeping both the mind and body in fighting shape. With exercise, the golden years can truly live up to their name.

As with any age group, the rules for senior exercise are straightforward: be consistent, start slow, and listen to your body. Remember Martha? Exercise transformed not just her body but her entire life. Whether it's walking, swimming, weightlifting, or even sprinting, find an activity that brings you joy and makes you feel alive.

The later chapters of our life book are yet to be written, and they can be as dynamic and fulfilling as any other stage of life. In fact, with the wisdom that comes with age, they could very well be your best chapters yet. Age

is just a number, but quality of life is a choice. Make the choice to move, to live, and to thrive.

So, here's to strong bones, flexible joints, and a beating heart that keeps pace with your grandkids. The time to start is now. Because remember, it's not about adding years to your life, but life to your years.

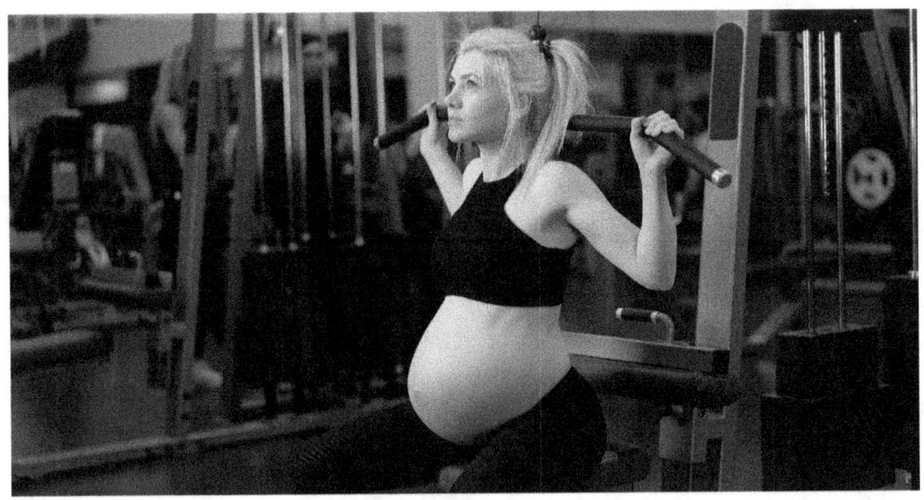

## Chapter 17:

### Exercise During Pregnancy

**"From Baby Bumps to Baby Jumps: The Fit Mama's Guide"**

Picture Serena Williams—tennis icon, entrepreneur, and a mother. Now cast your mind back to when she won the Australian Open while *eight weeks pregnant*. It was a ground-breaking moment that shattered conventional notions surrounding exercise and pregnancy. The story delivers a compelling message: Pregnancy does not spell the end of physical fitness. If anything, maintaining an exercise regimen can bring about a smoother pregnancy, faster recovery, and a host of benefits for both mom and baby.

**The Importance of Exercise During Pregnancy**

Staying active during pregnancy isn't just good for you—it's beneficial for your growing little one too. Regular exercise helps manage weight gain, improves mood, and can lead to easier labor and quicker postpartum recovery.

**Real-life Anecdote:** Emily's Transformation

Meet Emily, a first-time mom-to-be who initially shied away from exercise, fearing it could harm her baby. She was soon plagued by backaches, mood swings, and lethargy. On her doctor's advice, Emily incorporated moderate exercise into her routine. The result? Not only did her physical symptoms alleviate, but she also reported a boost in mental well-being. When her big day came, Emily's labor was relatively swift and she attributes her resilience and stamina to her fitness routine.

## Types of Exercises Suitable for Pregnancy

1. **Aerobic Exercise:** Swimming and walking are low-impact and effective.

2. **Strength Training:** Focus on light weights and high repetitions, avoiding heavy lifting and lying flat on your back.

3. **Flexibility and Relaxation:** Yoga and stretching can be excellent, but avoid hot yoga and deep twists.

## Daily Tasks and Training Program

*Daily Task 1:* **Hydration Monitoring**: Keep a water bottle handy and aim to consume at least 8 cups of water daily.

*Daily Task 2:* **Body Check:** Before and after exercises, assess how your body feels. Any discomfort should be a signal to modify or skip certain exercises.

## Training Program:

- **Week 1**: Begin with low-impact aerobic exercises. Aim for a 15-minute walk, 3 days a week.

- **Week 2:** Add body-weight exercises like squats and lunges. Aim for 2 sets of 10 reps twice a week.
- **Week 3:** Incorporate a basic stretching or pregnancy yoga routine for 15 minutes, 3 times a week.
- **Week 4:** Mix it up. Alternate between aerobic exercises and strength training, adding in flexibility routines whenever possible.

## Actionable Strategies

1. **Consult Your Doctor:** Before starting any exercise program, get clearance from your healthcare provider.
2. **Listen to Your Body:** Pregnancy is not the time to push through pain. If something feels off, stop immediately.
3. **Involve Your Partner:** Whether it's going for a walk or doing a home workout, involve your partner to make the exercise more enjoyable and motivating.

**Food for Thought:** The Mind-Body Connection

There's another reason why exercise during pregnancy is so vital —the mental health benefits. The endorphins released during exercise can combat pregnancy-related depression and anxiety. Moreover, the physical strength you build prepares you mentally for labor, enhancing the profound connection between mind and body.

## Summary

If Serena Williams can triumph at the Australian Open during her first trimester, you can certainly include some level of fitness in your nine-month journey. Exercise during pregnancy is not just about staving off weight gain; it's about building stamina for labor, boosting your mood, enhancing your resilience, and fostering a healthy environment for your unborn child.

Like Emily, you too can transform your pregnancy journey through the right kind of exercise, carefully tailored to each trimester and individual needs. Always remember to consult your healthcare provider and listen keenly to what your body tells you. You're not just eating for two; you're also *moving* for two, a notion that comes with its own set of responsibilities and rewards.

The journey of motherhood begins long before you hold your baby in your arms. It begins with taking care of yourself in a way that benefits both you and the new life growing inside you. So put on those maternity leggings, tie those shoelaces, and embrace the wonderful journey ahead. After all, a fit mama is often a happy mama, and a happy mama sets the stage for a happy, healthy baby.

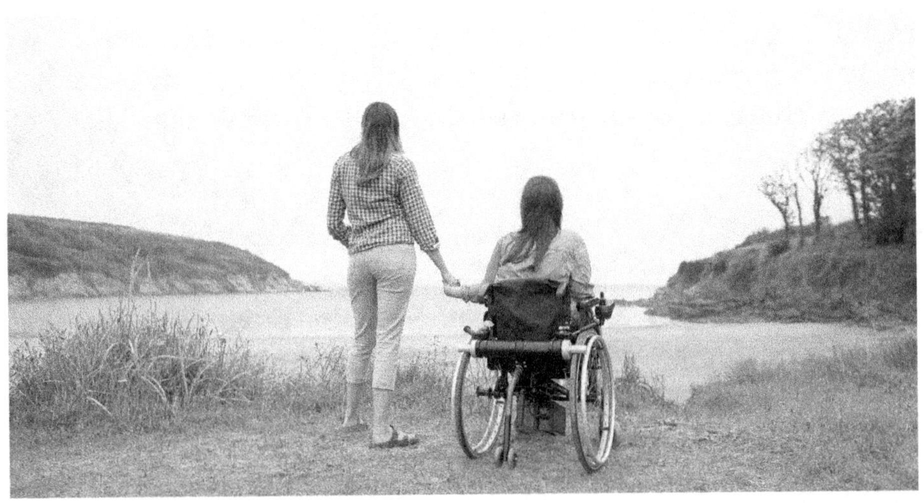

## Chapter 18:

## Adaptive Exercise for Disabilities

**"Breaking Barriers, One Rep at a Time"**

If you've ever been inspired by a story of human strength and resilience, prepare to add another to your list: that of Nick Vujicic. Born without arms or legs, Nick faces life challenges that most of us can hardly imagine. Yet, he is a motivational speaker, author, and swimmer who has taught the world that limitations are merely obstacles waiting to be overcome.

Nick's story isn't just an example of human tenacity; it's a powerful testament to how adaptive exercise can transform lives, even when faced with severe disabilities. Let's delve into this critical subject and explore how you, too, can overcome barriers through adaptive exercise.

**The Importance of Adaptive Exercise**

The benefits of regular exercise—enhanced mood, better health, increased longevity—are well-established. But what if you have mobility issues, chronic pain, or other disabilities? Does this mean exercise is off the table? Absolutely not. Adaptive exercise makes physical activity accessible to everyone, regardless of their limitations.

## Real-life Anecdote: Sarah's Journey

Sarah, who is wheelchair-bound due to cerebral palsy, had always considered gyms an alien world. That changed when she met an adaptive fitness trainer who designed a program focused on her abilities rather than disabilities. Within months, she found herself doing wheelchair sprints, weightlifting, and even yoga. Sarah's newfound strength did more than boost her physical abilities; **it** also transformed her self-esteem and opened doors to a community she never thought she'd be part of.

## Types of Adaptive Exercises

1. **Cardiovascular Training**: Activities like wheelchair sprints, swimming, or hand cycling improve cardiovascular health.

2. **Strength Training**: Using resistance bands, modified weightlifting equipment, or bodyweight exercises to build muscle.

3. **Flexibility Exercises**: Stretching and yoga can be adapted to various levels of mobility and can significantly improve range of motion.

## Daily Tasks and Training Program

*Daily Task 1*: **Breathing Exercises**: Spend at least 5 minutes focusing on your breath, which not only aids in relaxation but also prepares your lungs for exercise.

*Daily Task 2:* **Daily Mobility Check:** Move each joint as far as comfortably possible to understand your body's range for the day.

## Training Program:

- **Week 1:** Introduce yourself to cardiovascular exercises like arm-cycling or wheelchair sprints. Start with 10 minutes, 3 times a week.

- **Week 2:** Incorporate resistance training using bands or light weights, focusing on two muscle groups a week.

- **Week 3:** Add stretching exercises twice a week, each session lasting 15-20 minutes.

- **Week 4:** Evaluate your progress and adjust your routine based on your improvements and comfort levels.

## Actionable Strategies

1. **Consult Medical Professionals**: Before embarking on an adaptive exercise program, consult your doctor and preferably work with an adaptive fitness trainer.

2. **Customize, Don't Compromise:** Every exercise can be modified to suit your abilities. Don't settle for a one-size-fits-all approach.

3. **Community Involvement:** Join adaptive sports teams or online communities to stay motivated.

**Food for Thought:** Exercise is Empowerment

Adaptive exercise isn't merely a matter of physical well-being; it's an empowering tool that breaks down societal barriers and stereotypes. Each push, pull, or pedal is a testament to what people with disabilities can achieve—far beyond what society often expects from them.

## Summary

From Nick Vujicic's motivational speeches to Sarah's wheelchair sprints, we see that physical limitations don't have to limit your potential for a fulfilling, active life. Adaptive exercise offers a realm of possibilities for enhancing your health, boosting your confidence, and enriching your life in a myriad of ways.

As we've explored, the key steps include consulting with medical professionals, engaging with a specialized trainer, and employing a range of adaptive exercises from cardiovascular activities to strength training and flexibility exercises.

While society is catching up to the reality that individuals with disabilities have every right and ability to be as active as anyone else, you don't have to wait. With the right approach and community support, you can jump right into an adaptive exercise routine tailored for you.

The ball is in your court. Will you let societal norms define your limitations, or will you seize the empowering tools of adaptive exercise to carve out your own narrative of strength, resilience, and boundless potential? Remember, your limitations are often more mental than physical. Break those mental barriers, and there's no telling how far you can go. Exercise, after all, is a universal right, not a selective privilege. So gear up, get out there, and show the world what you're made of!

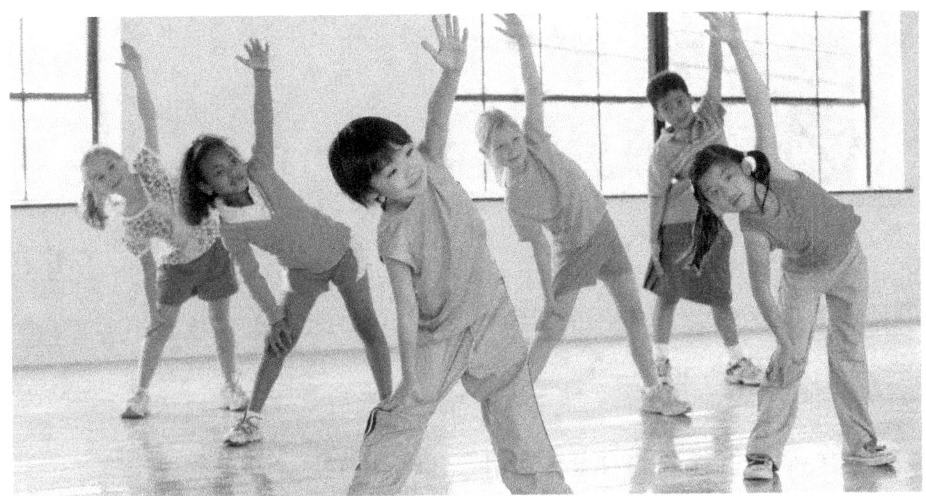

*Chapter 19:*

*Fitness for Kids*

## "Unlocking a Lifetime of Health: Play Today, Strong Tomorrow"

When we talk about childhood memories, we often reminisce about playground adventures, exhilarating bike rides, and games of tag that seemed as if they'd never end. But let's be real—today's children are far more likely to be engrossed in an iPad game than a game of hide-and-seek. While technology has brought numerous benefits, it's time we reintroduce the timeless treasure of physical activity into the lives of our children.

How about we kick things off with a compelling story? Enter Usain Bolt, the Jamaican sprinter nicknamed "Lightning Bolt." His Olympic gold medals and world records are legendary, but the seeds of his athleticism were sown in the sprint races he'd run as a child in rural Jamaica. No fancy gadgets, no state-of-the-art gym—just an open field and a passion for running. Bolt's journey is a vivid illustration that fostering fitness in childhood can lead to life-altering experiences later on.

## Why Fitness Matters for Kids

Childhood is the formative phase for instilling habits that last a lifetime. Physical fitness in childhood not only boosts physical health but also augments mental and emotional well-being. Regular exercise for kids improves focus, memory, and even academic performance.

**Real-life Anecdote:** Timmy's Transformation

Timmy, a 10-year-old boy, was on the verge of obesity and spent hours playing video games. His parents decided to make a change and enrolled him in a children's soccer program. Initially resistant, Timmy soon found himself enjoying not just the game but the newfound friendship and teamwork. Within a year, he was healthier, happier, and more confident.

## Types of Physical Activities for Kids

1. **Outdoor Games:** Soccer, basketball, or simple games like tag or duck-duck-goose.

2. **Indoor Activities:** Dance, gymnastics, or obstacle courses crafted with cushions and furniture.

3. **Family Outings:** Nature walks, cycling, or paddleboarding to involve the whole family in fitness.

## Daily Tasks and Training Program

*Daily Task 1:* **Screen Time Limit:** Limit screen time to one hour a day, encouraging kids to engage in physical activities.

*Daily Task 2:* **Healthy Snacks:** Replace chips or cookies with fruits or nuts to keep energy levels high.

## Training Program for the Week:

- **Monday:** Outdoor team sport like soccer or baseball (30 minutes)
- **Tuesday:** Family bike ride (20 minutes)
- **Wednesday:** Indoor obstacle course or hide-and-seek (30 minutes)
- **Thursday:** Nature walk or hiking (40 minutes)
- **Friday:** Dance or gymnastics class (30 minutes)
- **Saturday and Sunday:** Free play and family activity (45 minutes each day)

## Actionable Strategies

1. **Make It Fun:** Fitness for kids shouldn't feel like a chore. Make activities fun and engaging.
2. **Be a Role Model:** Children are more likely to be active if they see their parents setting an example.
3. **Encourage but Don't Push:** It's vital to encourage children but not force them into activities they do not enjoy.

**Food for Thought:** The Power of Choice

Allowing children to choose the type of physical activity they enjoy can be empowering and foster a lifelong love for fitness. Timmy didn't discover his love for soccer until he was given the chance to try it. And as Usain Bolt shows, who knows where such choices might lead?

## Summary

We need to revert to the roots of playful exercise when Xboxes didn't exist, and joy was derived from physical games that kept us active and healthy. As Usain Bolt's story teaches us, the formative years can be a precursor to greatness, and every child has within them a spark that needs just a bit of air to turn into a flame.

With Timmy, we see the transformational power of a lifestyle change, not only in terms of weight but in confidence, health, and happiness. Following simple daily tasks like screen time management and opting for healthier snacks can make a difference. Moreover, with a varied weekly training program, children can find what speaks to their hearts.

We've covered actionable strategies, from making fitness fun to leading by example and encouraging without pushing too hard. Remember, the goal isn't to raise the next Olympic champion; it's to instill healthy habits that will last a lifetime.

Fitness is not a sprint; it's a marathon, and the race begins in childhood. So let's ensure our kids have the most fun, enriching, and healthiest start to their lifelong journey of well-being. Because as it turns out, these little changes today can bring monumental benefits tomorrow, creating not just a stronger child but also a stronger future.

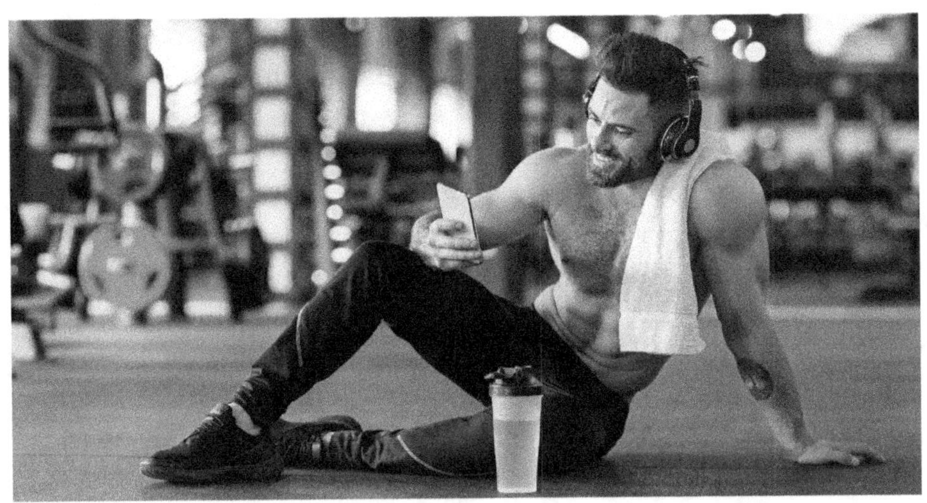

*Chapter 20:*

*The Role of Recovery*

**"Rest Is Not Laziness; It's Your Secret Weapon"**

"I'll sleep when I'm dead!" How many times have you heard this phrase in the gym, or perhaps even said it yourself? But what if I told you that taking time to recover could actually make you more fit, stronger, and even extend your life? Welcome to the often-overlooked world of recovery.

For our famous story, let's focus on none other than Michael Phelps, the most decorated Olympian of all time. While Phelps is famous for his rigorous training routines and unmatched commitment, he also prioritized recovery as an integral part of his training schedule. Think about it; his body couldn't possibly have withstood the intense hours of training without proper rest and recovery tactics like sleep, nutrition, and even 'cupping' therapy that became a talking point during the Olympics.

**Why Recovery Matters**

No matter how intense your workouts are, failing to give your body time to heal will lead to burnout, decreased performance, and a higher risk of injuries. The real gains aren't made during the workout but during the recovery period that follows.

**Real-life Anecdote:** Jane's Burnout

Jane was a fitness enthusiast who believed in pushing herself to the limits. She'd work out seven days a week, often doing double sessions. Initially, she saw gains but then hit a plateau and started experiencing frequent injuries. A fitness coach introduced her to the importance of recovery, which transformed her training and her life. She started making more significant gains in less time and with fewer injuries.

**The Facets of Recovery**

1. **Sleep:** The ultimate recovery tool. Lack of sleep can lead to poor performance, higher injury risks, and even chronic conditions like obesity and diabetes.

2. **Nutrition:** Your body needs fuel to repair itself. Proper nutrition is crucial for effective recovery.

3. **Active Recovery:** Activities like walking, swimming, or yoga that are less intense but still keep the body moving.

**Daily Tasks and Training Program**

*Daily Task 1:* **Sleep**: Aim for at least 7-9 hours of sleep.

*Daily Task 2:* **Nutrition:** Consume a balanced meal with carbs, proteins, and healthy fats within two hours of your workout.

**Training Program for Recovery:**

- **Monday:** High-intensity workout
- **Tuesday:** Active recovery—yoga or a 30-minute walk
- **Wednesday:** Strength training
- **Thursday:** Active recovery—swimming or cycling
- **Friday:** Cardio and HIIT
- **Saturday:** Complete rest or meditation
- **Sunday:** Fun physical activity of your choice

## Actionable Strategies

1. **Listen to Your Body:** If you feel excessive fatigue, consider skipping a workout and focus on recovery.
2. **Hydration:** Staying hydrated aids in faster recovery. Aim for at least 8 glasses of water a day.
3. **Stretch and Warm-Up:** Never underestimate the power of a good stretch or warm-up session before and after workouts.

**Food for Thought:** Mindfulness and Recovery

There's a growing body of research that indicates mindfulness and meditation can play a role in physical recovery. By lowering stress levels, you're also lowering cortisol levels, which aids in faster recovery and better performance.

## Summary

Even the most decorated Olympian, Michael Phelps, would never have reached the pinnacle of his career without prioritizing recovery. From Jane's journey, we learn that more doesn't always mean better. Effective recovery strategies not only prevent injuries but also help you make significant gains, taking your fitness journey to the next level.

Sleep, nutrition, and active recovery are the three pillars that support an effective recovery strategy. A balanced approach, like the one laid out in our weekly training program, ensures that you give your body the rest it needs without completely stalling your physical activity.

We also examined actionable strategies like listening to your body, hydrating, and incorporating stretching and warm-up into your routine. These aren't just add-ons; they're essentials. In the realm of fitness, rest isn't an act of surrender but a strategic move towards greater strength and well-being.

If you've been pushing the pedal to the metal with your workouts, remember that the road to fitness is not a sprint; it's a marathon. And every marathon has its rest stops. These aren't there to slow you down; they exist to ensure you can go the distance. So the next time you think of skipping that day off or cutting your sleep short, remember that recovery isn't the enemy of progress; it's an essential part of it.

In your quest for becoming healthier and stronger, make recovery your secret weapon. And just like Michael Phelps, who knows what heights you might reach when you give your body the rest it deserves?

# PART V: BEYOND THE GYM

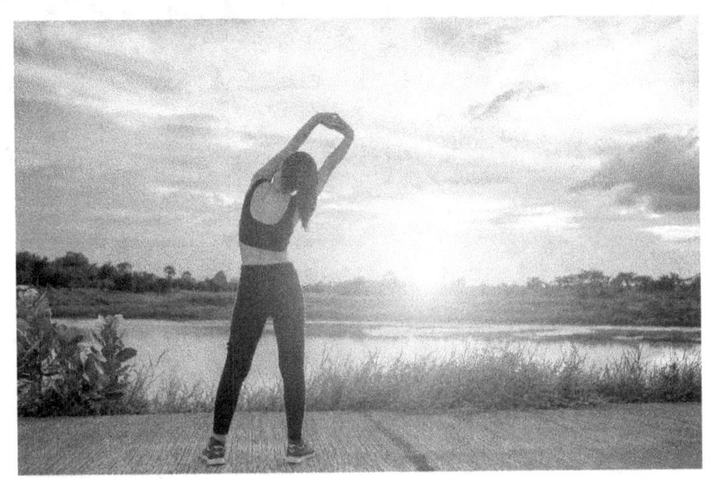

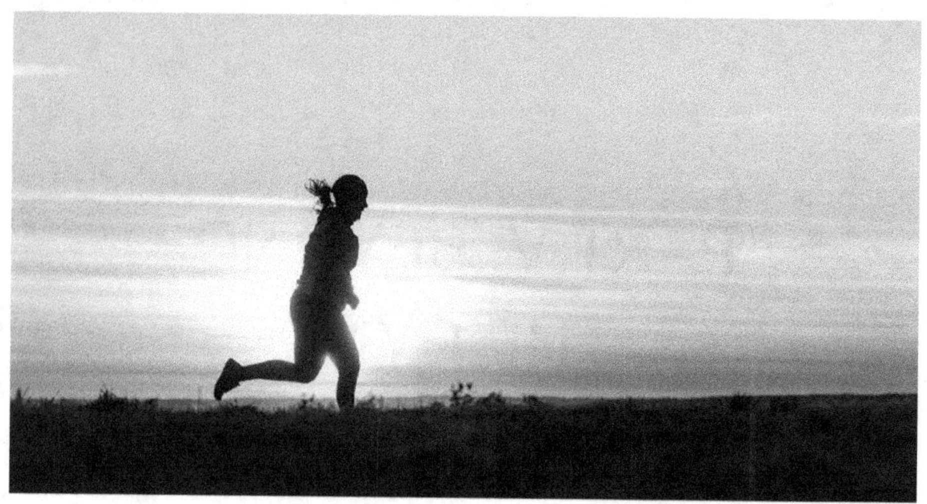

## Chapter 21:

## Fitness and Mental Health

**"Your Mind's Gym: The Secret Sanctuary for Mental Resilience"**

Imagine your brain as a fortress. Now, what if I told you that exercise is one of the strongest pillars holding up that fortress? Surprising, isn't it? Often, the focus of fitness is geared toward sculpting abs or building biceps, but the impact goes far beyond the physical—straight into the realms of mental and emotional well-being.

For our celebrity insight, let's consider the transformational story of actress and singer Demi Lovato. After battling issues related to mental health for years, Lovato has often cited exercise as a significant tool in managing her well-being. From Brazilian jiu-jitsu to regular gym workouts, she's found that physical activity offers her both a mental escape and a powerful tool for maintaining her mental health.

**Why Fitness is a Mental Game-Changer**

Exercise has proven benefits for mental health, including

reduced symptoms of depression, lower stress levels, and improved memory and cognitive function.

**Real-life Anecdote:** Mark's Upliftment

Mark was battling severe depression and felt like he was spiraling. Prescription meds and therapy weren't giving him the relief he sought. On the suggestion of a friend, he took up jogging. Initially, it was a struggle, but as days turned into weeks, something amazing happened. His mood started lifting. He still continued his therapy and medication, but the added regimen of physical exercise seemed to be the missing puzzle piece in his mental health journey.

## The Mind-Body Connection Explained

1. **Endorphins:** Exercise releases these 'feel-good' hormones, which act as natural mood lifters.

2. **Stress Reduction:** Physical activity reduces levels of the body's stress hormones, like adrenaline and cortisol.

3. **Better Sleep:** Regular physical activity, especially aerobic exercise, helps you fall asleep faster and deepens your sleep.

## Daily Tasks and Training Program

*Daily Task 1:* **Mindfulness Moment:** Start your day with a five-minute mindfulness exercise to center yourself.

*Daily Task 2:* **End-of-Day Reflection:** Spend 10 minutes reflecting on what made you grateful today.

**Training Program for Mental Health:**

- **Monday:** Cardiovascular Exercise (30 minutes) + Meditation (10 minutes)
- **Tuesday:** Strength Training (30 minutes) + Journaling (10 minutes)
- **Wednesday:** Yoga (40 minutes)
- **Thursday:** Nature Walk (30 minutes) + Deep Breathing Exercises (10 minutes)
- **Friday:** Dance/Zumba (30 minutes) + Gratitude Exercise (10 minutes)
- **Saturday:** Rest or Light Activity + Visualizations (15 minutes)
- **Sunday:** Leisure Swim or Bike Ride (30 minutes) + Positive Affirmations (10 minutes)

## Actionable Strategies

1. **Consistency Over Intensity:** Aim for regular, moderate exercise rather than occasional bursts of high-intensity workouts.

2. **Social Support:** Involve friends or family in your fitness journey for mutual encouragement.

3. **Consult Professionals:** Before starting any new fitness regimen, consult with healthcare providers, especially if you're using exercise as a supplementary treatment for mental health issues.

**Food for Thought:** Is Fitness a Cure-All?

While the benefits of exercise for mental health are undeniable, it's not a silver bullet. Medical conditions like depression and anxiety often require a multi-faceted approach, including medication and psychotherapy. Exercise should be a complementary treatment, not a replacement.

## Summary

As we've seen through the inspiring stories of Demi Lovato and Mark, exercise isn't just for building muscles or improving physical endurance; it's a crucial component for enhancing mental wellness. With the release of endorphins, stress hormone reduction, and improvement in sleep quality, the merits extend well beyond the treadmill or yoga mat.

Our daily tasks and training program offer a balanced mix of physical exercise and mindfulness techniques aimed at boosting your mental health. Consistency, social support, and professional guidance are key to implementing these successfully.

And while exercise is a potent tool for combating mental health issues, it should be part of a broader, more comprehensive treatment plan. It's not the only answer but part of the solution.

The journey to peak physical and mental fitness is a marathon, not a sprint. As you build your body, don't forget to fortify the fortress of your mind. After all, what's a strong body if the pillar that holds it up—the mind—isn't equally robust?

So the next time you're lacing up your sneakers or rolling out your yoga mat, remember: you're not just sculpting your muscles; you're also molding a stronger, more resilient mind. And that's a workout worth investing in.

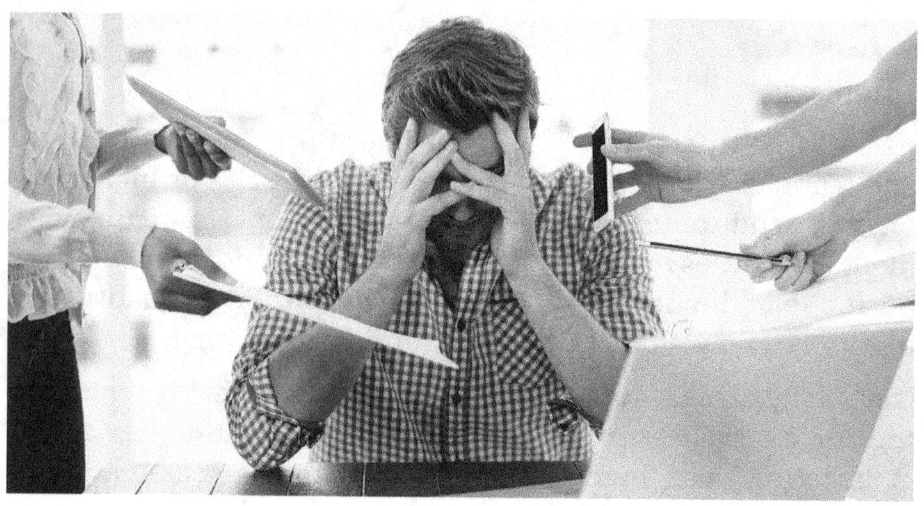

*Chapter 22:*

*Stress Management Techniques*

## "Shedding the Weight of Stress: Your Guide to Lightening the Load"

Picture this: a jigsaw puzzle with thousands of pieces, scattered and disorganized. Now, imagine that this puzzle represents your life. The secret to solving it? Managing stress effectively. In today's fast-paced world, stress is as unavoidable as traffic during rush hour. However, the key to a healthier, stronger you might lie in how well you handle life's little (or big) stressors.

Let's turn our attention to someone who mastered the art of stress management—Oprah Winfrey. From humble beginnings to being a media mogul, Oprah faced enormous stress and adversity. Her secret wasn't just resilience but also the practice of stress management techniques like meditation and journaling. Oprah has long advocated for taking out time each day to be present, mindful, and thankful.

## Stress: The Invisible Enemy

Just as lack of exercise or a poor diet can wreak havoc on your physical health, stress can be corrosive to both the body and mind.

**Real-life Anecdote:** Emily's Breaking Point

Emily was a high-powered executive, juggling work, family, and what she thought was a healthy lifestyle. But stress caught up with her, manifesting as crippling anxiety and weight gain. Her wake-up call was a stress-induced panic attack. With therapy and targeted stress management techniques, she turned her life around. Emily's case illustrates that even if you're doing everything else right, ignoring stress can derail your fitness journey.

**The Physiology of Stress**

1. **Cortisol Overload:** Stress triggers the release of cortisol, a hormone that, in high levels, can lead to weight gain and muscle breakdown.
2. **Fight or Flight:** The immediate response your body has to stress is to go into "fight or flight" mode, which is not sustainable long-term and can lead to fatigue and burnout.

**Daily Tasks and Training Program**

*Daily Task 1:* **Deep Breathing:** Start your day with 5 minutes of deep breathing to center your thoughts.

*Daily Task 2:* **Daily Gratitude:** Before bed, list three things you are grateful for.

## Training Program for Stress Management:

- **Monday:** Cardio workout (30 minutes) + Progressive Muscle Relaxation (PMR) technique (10 minutes)

- **Tuesday:** Yoga (30 minutes) + Journaling (15 minutes)

- **Wednesday:** Nature walk (30 minutes) + Mindfulness Meditation (10 minutes)

- **Thursday:** Pilates (30 minutes) + Visualization Exercise (10 minutes)

- **Friday:** Dancing (30 minutes) + Simple Breathing Exercises (5 minutes)

- **Saturday:** Free time/Rest + Affirmations (5 minutes)

- **Sunday:** Leisure activity + Guided Imagery Exercise (10 minutes)

## Actionable Strategies

1. **Identify Stress Triggers:** Make a list of things or situations that trigger stress. Awareness is the first step towards control.

2. **Boundaries:** Don't be afraid to say 'no' or to take time out for self-care.

3. **Seek Professional Help:** When stress becomes unmanageable, consult professionals like psychologists or counselors.

**Food for Thought:** Is All Stress Bad?

It's worth mentioning that not all stress is harmful. "Eustress," or positive stress, can actually be a motivating force. The key is to manage and balance stress effectively so that it doesn't evolve into distress, which is harmful.

## Summary

Stress, often overlooked, is as impactful on your wellness as any physical factor. Through the lens of Oprah's life and Emily's experience, we recognize the essential role of stress management in the pursuit of a healthier, stronger you.

From understanding the physiology of stress to following a weekly training program, you have a road map to manage stress effectively. Techniques like Deep Breathing, Progressive Muscle Relaxation, and Mindfulness Meditation aren't just buzzwords; they're practical tools you can use every day.

Lastly, while identifying stress triggers and setting boundaries are actionable steps, seeking professional guidance is advisable for persistent stress issues.

Remember, solving the jigsaw puzzle of life becomes easier when you know how to manage the pieces effectively. It's not just about handling what life throws at you, but also about equipping yourself with the skills to catch it, analyze it, and throw it back with grace.

By incorporating these stress management techniques into your daily routine, you're not just working towards a fitter body but also a more resilient mind. And that's a level of fitness worth striving for.

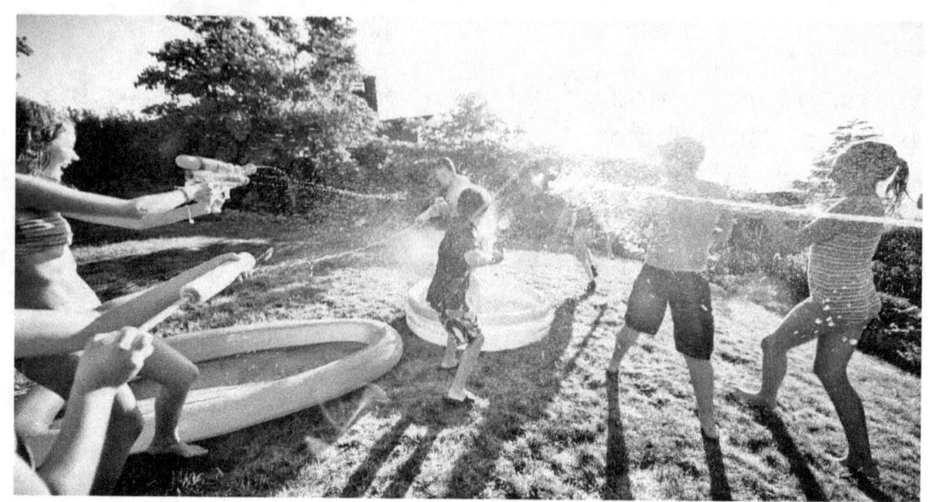

## Chapter 23:

## The Benefits of Outdoor Activities

**"Take a Breath of Fresh Air: Your Passport to Physical and Mental Fitness"**

You don't need an exclusive gym membership or the latest fitness gadgets to sculpt your body and elevate your mind. Nature itself can be your gym, your therapist, and your muse, all rolled into one. But don't just take my word for it—let's look at the fascinating story of celebrated author and naturalist, Henry David Thoreau. He eschewed conventional society for two years, opting to live in the woods. His experience, which he eloquently describes in "Walden," extols the virtues of being close to nature for physical and emotional well-being.

**The 'Natural' Way to Get Fit**

Remember climbing trees, running barefoot, and feeling the wind in your hair as a child? Back then, exercise wasn't a chore; it was a byproduct of outdoor fun.

Real-life Anecdote: Sarah's Adventure

Sarah was never a gym person. The treadmill bored her, and lifting weights felt like a punishment. She then discovered trail running. Something magical happened in the great outdoors—exercise didn't feel like "exercise" anymore. Sarah lost weight, her mood improved, and she even completed a half-marathon on rugged terrain!

## The Science Behind Outdoor Fitness

1. **Vitamin D Boost:** Exposing your skin to sunlight helps you produce vitamin D, vital for bone health and immune function.

2. **Mental Clarity:** Nature can help reduce mental fatigue by relaxing and restoring the mind.

3. **Oxygen and Air Quality:** Fresh air can boost your intake of oxygen, helping to increase the serotonin levels in your body, making you feel happier and more relaxed.

## Daily Tasks and Training Program

*Daily Task 1:* **Morning Light:** Spend at least 10 minutes in natural sunlight every morning.

*Daily Task 2:* **Evening Unwind:** Take a 20-minute walk outside every evening.

## Training Program for Outdoor Activities:

- **Monday:** Hiking (1 hour) + Nature Journaling (10 minutes)

- **Tuesday:** Outdoor Cycling (30 minutes) + Bird Watching (20 minutes)
- **Wednesday:** Open Water Swimming (20 minutes) + Meditation by the Water (10 minutes)
- **Thursday:** Trail Running (30 minutes) + Forest Bathing (20 minutes)
- **Friday:** Kayaking (1 hour)
- **Saturday:** Rest + Outdoor Picnic and Leisure Time (2 hours)
- **Sunday:** Outdoor Yoga (45 minutes) + Nature Photography (1 hour)

## Actionable Strategies

1. **Start Small:** If you're new to outdoor activities, start with short, manageable timeframes and then gradually increase.
2. **Safety First:** Always ensure you have adequate safety measures in place—whether it's a lifejacket for kayaking or a map for hiking.
3. **Be Present:** Leave your gadgets behind or put them on silent. The point is to connect with nature, not Wi-Fi.

**Food for Thought**: Balancing Outdoor and Indoor Activities

While outdoor activities are incredible for mental and physical health, they aren't a complete substitute for a balanced, indoor fitness routine. Certain muscle groups may not get adequately targeted, and weather conditions can disrupt your routine.

## Summary

Henry David Thoreau's sojourn into the woods wasn't just a

poetic escapade; it was a declaration of the essential role nature plays in our physical and mental well-being. Similarly, Sarah's transformation through trail running illustrates that nature can be a compelling and enjoyable avenue for fitness.

Our bodies and minds are designed to resonate with the natural world. The sunlight kissing your skin isn't just a poetic encounter; it's a Vitamin D boost. The wind rushing past you doesn't just feel exhilarating; it's also enhancing your mood and oxygenating your cells.

The daily tasks and training programs provided are more than just a set of activities; they're an invitation to reconnect with nature and, in doing so, reconnect with yourself. Whether it's hiking, kayaking, or simply strolling through a forest, the great outdoors is a treasure trove of fitness opportunities.

So, the next time you're about to hit 'Start' on that treadmill, consider hitting the trail instead. As you venture out, remember that every step taken on the soil is a step closer to your roots, and every breath of fresh air is a sigh of relief for your soul.

When you engage in outdoor activities, you're not just building muscle or losing weight; you're becoming one with nature, and perhaps, rediscovering a piece of yourself that got lost in the hustle and bustle of modern life. Now that's what I call holistic fitness!

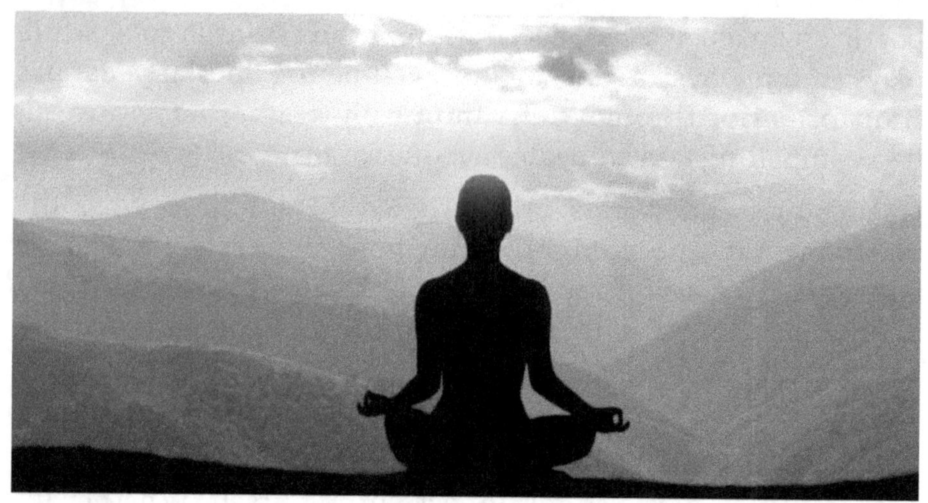

*Chapter 24:*

*Yoga and Mindfulness*

## "Unlock the Power of Mind-Body Connection for Total Fitness"

Think of Jennifer Aniston, a Hollywood A-lister who has stayed fit and fabulous for decades. One of her secret weapons? Yoga and mindfulness. Aniston's practice isn't just about looking great on the red carpet; it's about nurturing her mental, emotional, and spiritual well-being. Let's delve into the transformative world of yoga and mindfulness, and discover how you can cultivate your own personal well-being through this ancient practice.

## The Union of Mind and Body

Yoga isn't just a series of poses; it's a holistic practice that unites the mind, body, and spirit. Similarly, mindfulness isn't about sitting in a Zen-like state; it's about being fully present in whatever you're doing.

**Real-life Anecdote: Tim's Transformation**

Tim was a corporate executive dealing with chronic back pain and mounting stress. His doctor prescribed medications, but they only masked the symptoms. Tim turned to yoga and mindfulness as a last resort. The results were astounding. Not only did his back pain subside, but his stress levels plummeted. Even his colleagues noticed a change in his demeanor; he was calmer, more focused, and happier.

**The Science of Yoga and Mindfulness**

**Yoga:**

1. **Flexibility:** It improves flexibility by stretching and relaxing the muscles.
2. **Strength:** Yoga uses body weight to build muscle tone.
3. **Stress Reduction:** It helps reduce cortisol levels, aiding in stress management.

**Mindfulness:**

1. **Mental Clarity:** Mindfulness helps in reducing mental chatter.
2. **Emotional Regulation:** Being mindful helps you manage your emotional responses better.
3. **Enhanced Focus:** Regular mindfulness practice can improve your concentration.

**Daily Tasks and Training Program**

*Daily Task 1*: Spend at least 5 minutes in a meditative state every morning.

***Daily Task 2:*** Do a 20-minute yoga routine that focuses on your problem areas—be it flexibility, strength, or relaxation.

## Training Program:

- **Monday:** Vinyasa Yoga (40 minutes) + Mindfulness Breathing (5 minutes)
- **Tuesday:** Hatha Yoga for Strength (35 minutes) + Body Scan Meditation (10 minutes)
- **Wednesday:** Restorative Yoga (30 minutes) + Loving-kindness Meditation (5 minutes)
- **Thursday:** Power Yoga (45 minutes) + Mindful Eating (15 minutes)
- **Friday:** Yin Yoga for Flexibility (40 minutes) + Silent Walking Meditation (10 minutes)
- **Saturday:** Kundalini Yoga (50 minutes) + Mindful Journaling (10 minutes)
- **Sunday:** Free-form Yoga (20 minutes) + Mindful Nature Walk (30 minutes)

## Actionable Strategies

1. Consistency is Key: Both yoga and mindfulness require regular practice for noticeable results.

2. Personalization: Customize your practice to suit your needs. Yoga is not one-size-fits-all.

3. Seek Guidance: Especially if you're a beginner, don't hesitate to take professional help to ensure you're doing it right.

**Food for Thought:** Yoga and Mindfulness Beyond the Mat

Both practices offer benefits that extend well beyond your yoga mat. How can you take the principles of mindfulness and apply them to your daily life? For instance, can you eat mindfully, appreciating every bite? Can you perform your work tasks with the same level of focused attention as a yoga pose?

## Summary

The stories of Jennifer Aniston and Tim reflect the broad spectrum of benefits that yoga and mindfulness offer. From physical fitness to mental clarity, these practices offer a holistic approach to well-being that is more relevant today than ever.

The science-backed explanations not only validate the effectiveness of yoga and mindfulness but also help you understand the mechanics behind the magic. This isn't just about 'feeling good'; it's about biological and psychological transformations that empower you for the challenges of daily life.

The daily tasks and training programs provided are designed to be comprehensive yet flexible. Just like yoga itself, these programs are adaptable to meet the unique needs of every individual. The actionable strategies aim to make this journey as smooth as possible for you.

Finally, the concept of taking yoga and mindfulness beyond the mat opens a whole new world of possibilities. This isn't just a fitness regimen; it's a lifestyle. The principles you practice on the mat can spill over into every aspect of your life, from how you work to how you interact with others.

So why wait? Embark on this incredible journey and experience the union of body, mind, and spirit. Yoga and mindfulness are not just 'activities' but a way of living—a path to a healthier, stronger, and more serene you.

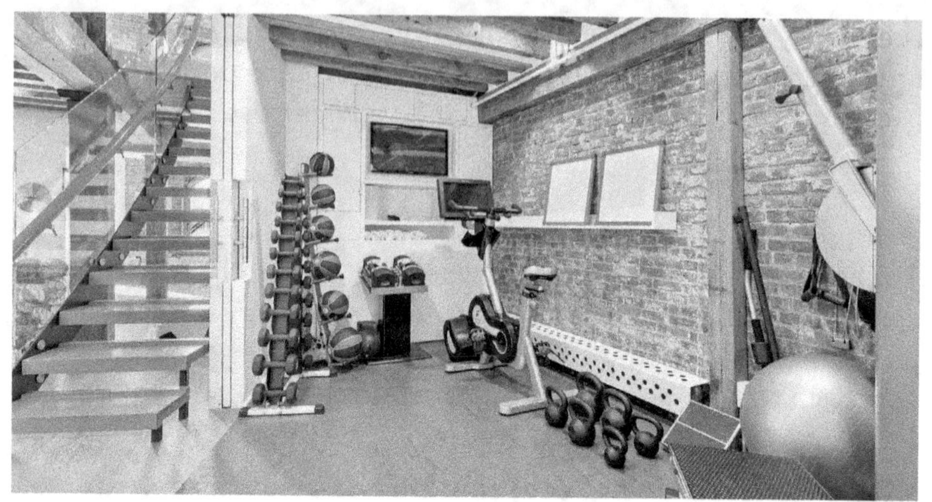

*Chapter 25:*

*Building a Home Gym*

## "The Ultimate Guide to Crafting Your Personal Fitness Sanctuary"

When you hear about home gyms, perhaps you envision Dwayne "The Rock" Johnson, one of the biggest action stars on the planet, lifting colossal weights in his state-of-the-art Iron Paradise. While most of us can't construct a multi-million-dollar fitness playground, the beauty is you don't have to. You can tailor a home gym to fit your space, budget, and fitness goals. If The Rock can build his dream gym, so can you!

## The What and Why of Home Gyms

**Real-life Anecdote:** Sarah's Success Story

Meet Sarah, a 35-year-old mother of two who works from home. With limited time and even less inclination to hit the public gym, she decided to set up a small workout corner in her garage. Within months, she lost 20 pounds, improved her cardiovascular health, and elevated her mental wellness.

## The Benefits of a Home Gym

1. **Convenience:** Exercise on your timetable, not the gym's.
2. **Customization:** Select equipment based on your goals.
3. **Privacy:** Work out without feeling self-conscious.

## The Essentials: Setting up a Home Gym

### Space

Identify a dedicated space that will serve as your home gym. It could be a spare bedroom, a section of the garage, or even a corner of your living room.

### Equipment

1. Cardio Machines: Treadmill, elliptical, or stationary bike.
2. Strength Equipment: Dumbbells, kettlebells, or resistance bands.
3. Accessories: Yoga mat, stability ball, and jump rope.

## Daily Tasks and Training Program

### Daily Tasks:

1. **Regular Maintenance:** Dust off the equipment and check for wear and tear.
2. **Equipment Rotation:** Switch out equipment every two weeks to prevent workout stagnation.

## Four-Week Training Program

- **Week 1:**
  - Monday: Treadmill - 20 minutes
  - Wednesday: Dumbbell workout - 3 sets of 10 reps
  - Friday: Yoga and stretching
- **Week 2:**
  - Monday: Elliptical - 25 minutes
  - Wednesday: Kettlebell workout - 3 sets of 8 reps
  - Friday: Resistance band exercises
- **Week 3:**
  - Monday: Cycling on stationary bike - 30 minutes
  - Wednesday: Dumbbell and kettlebell mixed workout
  - Friday: Yoga and stretching
- **Week 4:**
  - Monday: Treadmill HIIT - 20 minutes
  - Wednesday: Full-body strength workout
  - Friday: Yoga and mindfulness

## Actionable Strategies

1. **Start Small**: You don't need to buy everything at once.
2. **Quality over Quantity:** Invest in durable equipment that will last.
3. **Consult an Expert:** Speak with a fitness trainer for personalized advice on equipment and layout.

**Food for Thought:** Does the Perfect Home Gym Exist?

The notion of a "perfect" home gym is subjective. What works for a pro athlete may not be ideal for you. Your "perfect" gym is one that aligns with your fitness goals, budget, and available space. So, don't obsess over creating a picture-perfect setup. Instead, focus on building a functional space that makes you look forward to your workouts.

## Summary

The stories of Dwayne "The Rock" Johnson and Sarah exemplify the potential of home gyms—from luxurious setups to functional, budget-friendly spaces. But no matter the scale, all home gyms share common benefits: convenience, customization, and privacy.

Setting up a home gym might seem daunting, but breaking it down into manageable tasks makes it easier. Start by identifying your available space, and then choose the equipment that matches your fitness goals. Following a training program can help you get the most out of your investment.

The actionable strategies offer a roadmap to a successful home gym setup, emphasizing the importance of starting small, focusing on quality, and seeking expert advice.

The concept of the 'perfect' home gym is fluid and personalized, so the most important thing is to build a space that inspires you to get fit and stay that way.

So, roll up your sleeves, get out your tools, and start building your home gym. Whether it's a humble corner with basic equipment or an expansive haven filled with high-tech gadgets, remember that the best gym is the one you'll actually use. With a little effort and planning, you can create a home gym that sets you up for a lifetime of health and well-being.

# PART VI: ROADBLOCKS AND SOLUTIONS

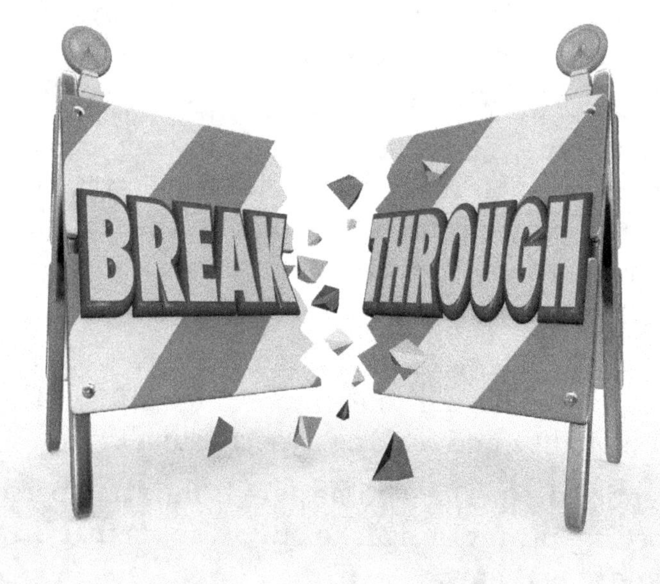

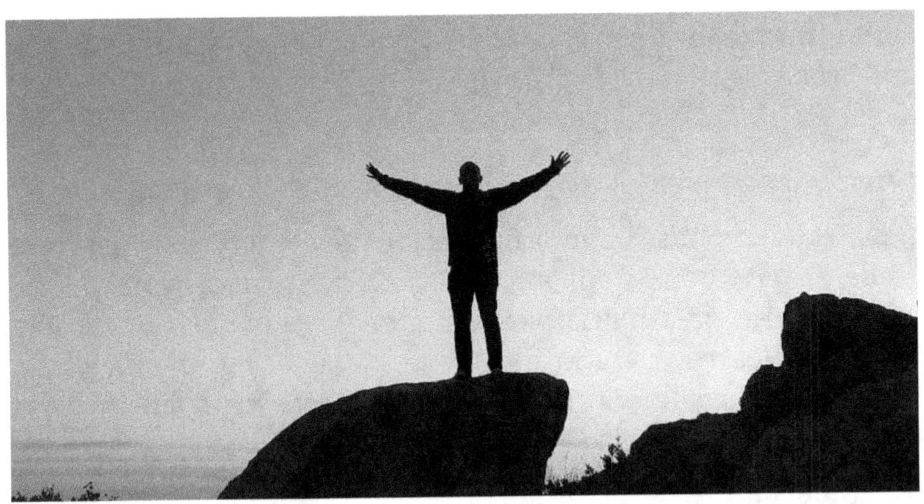

*Chapter 26:*

*Overcoming Plateaus*

## "The Art of Smashing Through the Fitness Ceiling"

Imagine you're cruising down a highway at 60 mph. Everything seems smooth, but suddenly you hit traffic. No matter how hard you push on the gas, you're stuck. This frustrating scenario mirrors what many face in their fitness journey—a plateau. Even legends like Arnold Schwarzenegger have hit plateaus, only to blast through them and achieve iconic physiques. Let's dive in and discover how you too can overcome your fitness roadblocks.

## The Plateau Phenomenon

**Real-life Anecdote:** Emily's Experience

Emily, a 30-year-old finance manager, had been working out for years. She lost weight, toned her muscles, but then progress came to a screeching halt. Despite following the same regimen, her improvements just stopped. Sounds familiar? Emily's story is not unique, but her solution was. She revamped her routine and broke free from her plateau.

## What is a Plateau?

A plateau is a phase in your fitness journey where your progress stalls despite consistent effort. It can happen in weight loss, muscle gain, or athletic performance. Your body, remarkably adaptive, learns to perform your routine more efficiently, burning fewer calories or minimizing muscle engagement.

## Arnold Schwarzenegger's Story

Even the "Austrian Oak" Arnold Schwarzenegger faced plateaus. Early in his bodybuilding career, Arnold felt his progress had slowed. His solution? Changing his workout routine, implementing "shock" tactics, and focusing on his weaker areas. This helped him win Mr. Olympia titles and build one of the most iconic physiques in history.

## Daily Tasks and Training Program to Overcome Plateaus

## Daily Tasks:

1. **Track Progress:** Keep a workout log to measure your performance.
2. **Listen to Your Body:** Make a note of how you feel before, during, and after exercise.
3. **Nutritional Adjustment:** Review your caloric intake and macros.

## Four-Week Training Program to Beat Plateaus

- **Week 1:**

- Evaluate Weak Areas
- Revisit Basic Movements
- Incorporate Mobility Drills
- **Week 2:**
    - Introduce Variation
    - Different Exercise Equipment
    - Add Supersets or Drop Sets
- **Week 3:**
    - Intensify Workouts
    - Increase Weight or Resistance
    - Reduce Rest Periods
- **Week 4:**
    - Implement "Shock" Techniques
    - Adopt High-Intensity Interval Training (HIIT)
    - Include Plyometrics

## Actionable Strategies

1. **Identify the Plateau:** Sometimes you might think you've hit a plateau when you're actually still progressing. Use metrics to confirm.

2. **Consult a Coach:** Sometimes an external perspective can provide fresh insights into what you're doing right or wrong.

3. **Nutritional Review:** Often a plateau can be the result of a diet that hasn't adapted to your new body metrics.

4. **Rest and Recover:** Maybe your plateau is a sign of overtraining. Proper rest might be all you need.

**Food for Thought:** The Plateau as a Friend?

What if we see the plateau not as an enemy, but a friend signaling us to evolve? A plateau can serve as a checkpoint—a pause to reflect, adapt, and shoot for higher goals.

## Summary

Hitting a plateau can be both frustrating and confusing, but it's a natural part of any fitness journey. Take Arnold Schwarzenegger for example; he didn't become a bodybuilding legend by remaining static. He busted through his plateaus by being innovative and relentless in his approach.

To overcome your own plateau, it's essential to identify it first. Tools like a workout log can help you track your progress and pinpoint where things have stalled. Emily's anecdote illustrates how a plateau isn't a dead-end but rather a detour that can lead you to a more effective and engaging fitness journey.

A carefully designed training program can introduce the variation and intensity needed to shake things up and force your body to adapt. Consulting with a fitness coach can provide additional perspectives that you may have overlooked.

So the next time you find yourself stuck in a fitness rut, don't despair. See it as a signal from your body that it's time for a change. With smart strategies and a fresh mindset, you can break through that plateau and soar to new fitness heights. You have the tools, and you have the roadmap. Now get out there and break through that ceiling!

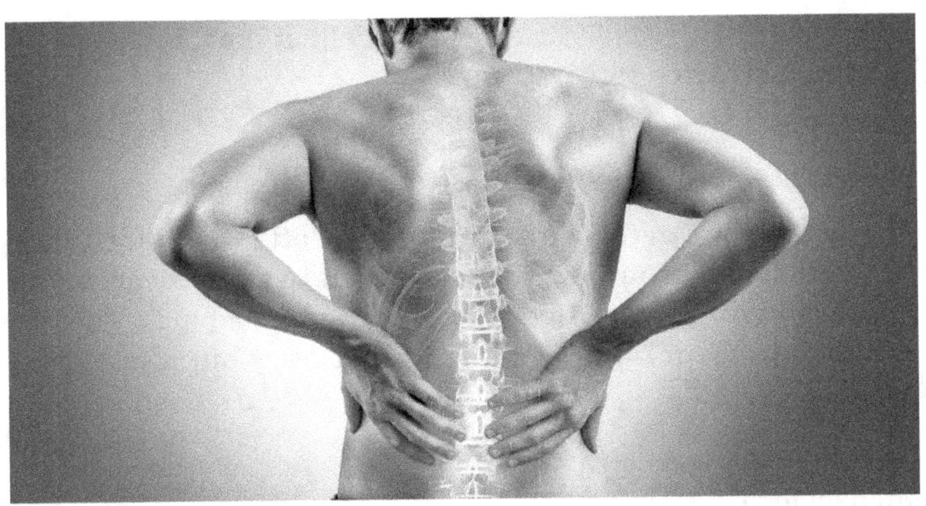

*Chapter 27:*

*Dealing with Injuries*

## "When Obstacles Turn into Opportunities"

Imagine being on the journey of your life, driving through a picturesque landscape, feeling invincible, and then you hit a roadblock—your car breaks down. Now, what? The same goes for fitness. You're making progress, lifting heavier, running faster, and then suddenly you're on the sidelines nursing an injury. A setback? Yes. But also an opportunity for growth. Just ask Michael Jordan.

## The Injury Challenge

### Real-life Anecdote: Sarah's Struggle

Sarah, a 26-year-old marketing executive, was a gym enthusiast who loved CrossFit. One unfortunate day, she twisted her ankle during a workout. Frustrated and disheartened, Sarah had to take a break. But she didn't let her injury define her. Instead, she took it as a challenge, educating herself about rehabilitation and building a smarter, safer routine.

## The Reality of Injuries

No matter how careful you are, injuries are often an unfortunate part of the fitness journey. They can be due to a variety of factors such as improper form, overtraining, or even bad luck. The key to handling them is not just physical recovery but also mental resilience.

## Michael Jordan's Lesson

Remember when Michael Jordan broke his foot in his second NBA season? People thought it might be the end of his career. But Jordan used his time off-court for rehabilitation and conditioning. Not only did he come back, but he also led the Chicago Bulls to multiple championships. His mindset? "Obstacles don't have to stop you. If you run into a wall, don't turn around and give up. Figure out how to climb it."

## Daily Tasks and Rehabilitation Program

### Daily Tasks:

1. **Initial Assessment**: Determine the severity of the injury. If needed, consult a medical professional.
2. **Active Recovery**: Gentle stretches and mobility work if permissible.
3. **Education**: Learn about your injury, so you can discuss it with your healthcare provider better.

## Four-Week Rehabilitation Program:

**Note:** Always consult a healthcare provider for a personalized rehabilitation program.

- **Week 1:**
    - Injury Assessment
    - Ice and Elevation
    - Gentle, Isometric Exercises
- **Week 2:**
    - Physical Therapy Consultation
    - Begin Mobility Exercises
    - Nutrition Assessment for Recovery
- **Week 3:**
    - Advanced Mobility Drills
    - Soft Tissue Manipulation (massage or foam rolling)
    - Incorporate Resistance Bands
- **Week 4:**
    - Return to Activity Assessment
    - Revisit Exercise Technique
    - Gradual Re-Introduction to Weight Training

## Actionable Strategies

1. **Medical Consultation:** The first step after an injury should always be to consult a medical professional for an accurate diagnosis and a rehabilitation program.

2. **Mindset Shift:** Treat your injury as a learning curve. Use the downtime to better understand your body and how to keep it injury-free.

3. **Active Recovery:** When permitted, engage in light exercise to facilitate recovery.

4. **Nutritional Support:** Your body will need particular nutrients to heal. Ensure your diet supports your recovery goals.

**Food for Thought:** The Gift in the Curse?

An injury can be a hidden blessing. It forces you to stop, reevaluate, and refine your fitness journey. Instead of seeing it as a hindrance, consider it a form of 'forced introspection,' a time to dive deep into understanding your body and its needs better.

**Summary**

Injuries are inevitable, but they don't define you or your fitness journey. What matters is how you respond to them. Sarah, confined by her twisted ankle, used her time to learn and grow, turning her setback into a comeback. Michael Jordan converted his injury into a championship-winning return.

You can do it too. Follow a structured rehabilitation program, seek professional guidance, and ensure your nutrition backs your recovery. Above all, remember that your mindset is a pivotal part of this journey. Embrace your injury as an opportunity to come back stronger, smarter, and more resilient than ever.

Injuries are not just roadblocks but also signposts, telling you to slow down, reevaluate, and course-correct. They can be frustrating, but they can also be enlightening. So the next time you find yourself nursing an injury, remember, it's not the end of the road, but a detour toward a more holistic, intelligent approach to fitness. A minor setback paves the way for a major comeback. So arm yourself with knowledge, brace yourself with determination, and set out to conquer your fitness journey anew.

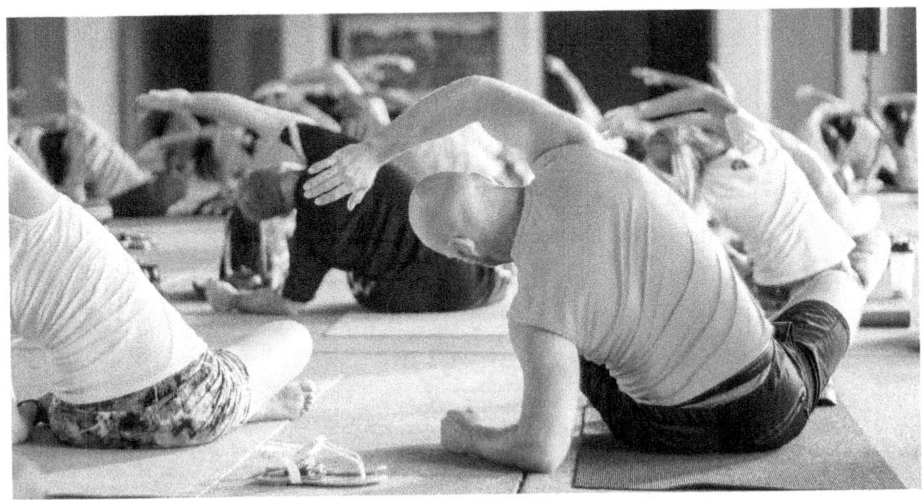

*Chapter 28:*

*Exercise and Chronic Illness*

## "The Extra Mile: When Fitness Conquers the Unconquerable"

In our journey through the world of fitness, we've covered several terrains. From the highs of achieving fitness milestones to the lows of injuries, we've learned that there's always a way **forward.** However, for some, the challenge is not just about hitting a plateau or overcoming a sprained ankle; it's about battling a constant internal storm—chronic illness.

## Your Fitness Journey, Tailored

**Real-life Anecdote:** Lisa's Triumph

Lisa, a spirited 32-year-old, was diagnosed with rheumatoid arthritis at the age of 25. For many, this might seem like a life sentence of immobility and pain. But not for Lisa. Instead of resigning herself to her fate, she chose to fight back with exercise, transforming her chronic condition from a dominating force to just another facet of her life.

## Chronic Illness: The Unseen Battle

Chronic illnesses, like diabetes, heart disease, and autoimmune disorders, can be life-altering. However, with the right approach and mindset, they don't have to dictate your life. Exercise, tailored to individual needs, can be a powerful tool against the debilitating effects of these conditions.

## A Celestial Role Model: Selena Gomez

Selena Gomez, the pop sensation and actress, was diagnosed with lupus, an autoimmune disease, in her early twenties. Instead of letting the illness overshadow her life, she used exercise as a means to cope, emphasizing its role in managing her symptoms and boosting her mental health. Gomez stands as a testament that with dedication, chronic illness can be managed and even incorporated into a holistic fitness journey.

## Daily Tasks and Training Program

### Daily Tasks:

1. **Self-Assessment:** Listen to your body. Recognize and respect its limits.
2. **Medication & Monitoring:** Ensure timely intake of medications and regular health check-ups.
3. **Light Activity:** Engage in light stretching or walking to keep the body active, even on rest days.

## Six-Week Training Program for Chronic Illness:

Note: Always consult a healthcare provider before starting any exercise regimen.

- **Week 1 & 2:**
    - **Aerobic Exercise:** Start with low-impact exercises like walking or cycling for 10-15 minutes a day.
    - **Strength Training:** Light resistance training using resistance bands or light weights.
- **Week 3 & 4:**
    - **Aerobic Exercise:** Increase duration to 20-25 minutes. Incorporate swimming if possible.
    - **Strength Training:** Gradually increase the weight or resistance while ensuring proper form.
- **Week 5 & 6:**
    - **Aerobic Exercise:** Aim for 30 minutes. Mix different forms of low-impact exercises.
    - **Strength Training:** Introduce more compound movements with adequate rest in between.

## Actionable Strategies

1. **Tailored Exercise Plan:** Recognize that your chronic condition is unique. Design a fitness plan that considers its specific challenges and requirements.
2. **Pace Yourself:** Start slow and listen to your body. Your progress might be slower than others, but it's progress nonetheless.
3. **Stay Informed:** Educate yourself about your illness. The more you know, the better equipped you'll be to navigate its challenges.

**Food for Thought:** Is Your Illness in Control, or Are You?

It's essential to remember that chronic illness is a part of you, but it isn't YOU. Like Lisa, who refused to let rheumatoid arthritis dominate her life, you too can reclaim control. Using exercise as a tool, you can mitigate symptoms, enhance well-being, and above all, remind yourself of your strength and resilience.

## Summary

Exercise and chronic illness might seem like strange bedfellows. Yet, time and time again, stories like Lisa's and Selena Gomez's prove that they can coexist, harmoniously and beneficially. The key lies in understanding your specific condition, tailoring your exercise regimen, and above all, cultivating a mindset of resilience.

Embracing exercise doesn't mean ignoring your illness. On the contrary, it means acknowledging it, understanding it, and then strategically using exercise to combat its adverse effects. After all, fitness isn't just about building muscles or endurance; it's about enhancing the overall quality of life. And for those battling chronic conditions, this quality can indeed be uplifted with the right fitness approach.

Remember, every step you take, every weight you lift, and every lap you swim isn't just a testament to your physical strength but a shoutout to your indomitable spirit. Your chronic illness may have introduced a new narrative to your life, but with exercise in your arsenal, you get to decide how this story unfolds.

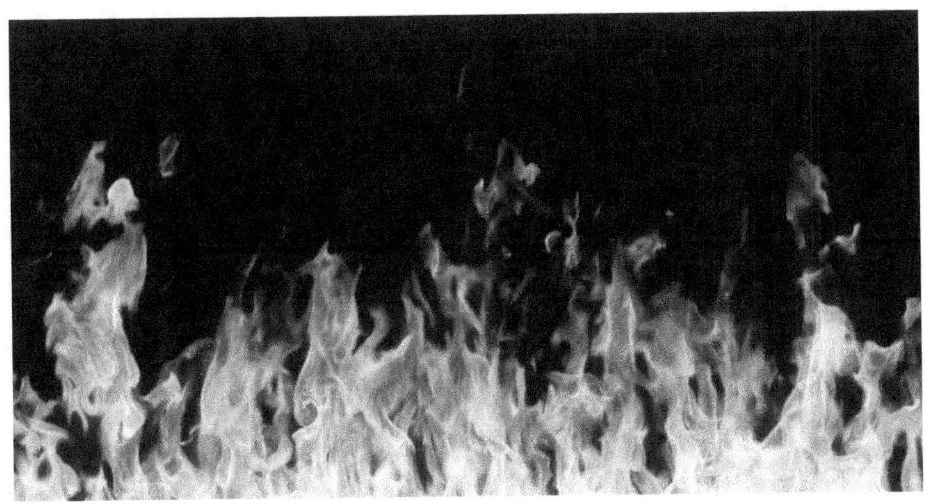

## Chapter 29:

## Motivation - Keeping the Fire Alive

*"It's not about having the skill to do something. It's about having the will, desire, and commitment to be your best."* - Robert Hernandez

For many, starting a fitness journey is a burst of energy, a newfound love. But like any relationship, there come times when the initial spark fades. The allure of a snooze button might overpower the morning run, or a busy schedule might push gym time to the sidelines. So, how do you keep the fire of motivation alive, especially when challenges seem insurmountable? Let's dive in.

**From a Single Step to a Marathon: Sarah's Journey**

Sarah was your average office worker. A sedentary lifestyle and the convenience of fast food had her tipping the scales. One day, she decided to change. The initial days were fantastic. Waking up early, eating clean, she was on top of the world. But three weeks in, the spark dimmed. Rainy mornings made her bed more inviting than the damp streets, and pizza won over salads.

Yet, she's now finished her third marathon. How?

## Motivation: It's Not One-Size-Fits-All

Every individual has a different motivation source. For some, it's about looking good for a special occasion. For others, it's health-driven. Finding and continuously reminding oneself of this 'why' is the key.

## Dwayne 'The Rock' Johnson: The Pillar of Consistency

The Rock, one of Hollywood's top earners and a former professional wrestler, swears by his gym routine. But even he has his days of struggle. His secret? He doesn't rely solely on motivation; he relies on discipline and remembers his humble beginnings and the reasons he started. By having a deep-rooted 'why' and coupling it with discipline, he ensures that he stays consistent.

## Daily Tasks and Training Program

## Daily Tasks:

1. **Visual Reminders:** Keep a photo or quote that resonates with your 'why' in places you often look - like your mirror or phone wallpaper.

2. **Track Your Progress:** Maintain a fitness diary. Jot down daily achievements, no matter how small.

3. **Stay Social:** Share milestones on social media or with close ones. The positive feedback loop can be a potent motivator.

## 4-Week Motivation Booster Program:

- **Week 1:** *Revisit Your Goals*
    - **Day 1-3:** Reflect on why you started. Write down three core reasons.
    - **Day 4-7:** Break down your main goal into mini-goals. Celebrate when you achieve them.
- **Week 2:** *Switch It Up*
    - **Day 1-3:** Try a new fitness activity or class.
    - **Day 4-7:** Introduce a new healthy recipe to your diet.
- **Week 3:** *Group Power*
    - **Day 1-3:** Work out with a friend or join a local fitness group.
    - **Day 4-7:** Participate in a group challenge or a community run.
- **Week 4:** *Reward System*
    - **Day 1-3:** Treat yourself (non-food) for every three consistent days of exercise.
    - **Day 4-7:** Reflect on the month's achievements and set goals for the next month.

**Actionable Strategies:**

1. **Stay Accountable:** Having a workout buddy can significantly enhance motivation. On days you feel low, they can be your push, and vice versa.

2. **Educate Yourself:** Read about fitness, understand the science behind exercises, and the benefits. The more you know, the more committed you become.

3. **Avoid Burnout:** Over-enthusiasm can lead to quick burnouts. Ensure rest days, and understand it's a marathon, not a sprint.

## Food for Thought: Is It Lack of Motivation or Fear of Failure?

Often, our demotivation stems from fear—fear of not achieving, fear of judgment. Understanding and acknowledging this fear can be the first step towards reigniting the motivational flame. Remember Sarah? Her dip came from the fear that she might never change, but once she recognized that, she found ways to conquer it, one run at a time.

## Summary:

Staying motivated through a fitness journey isn't about never having lows. It's about pushing through despite them. It's about remembering the 'why' when the 'how' becomes challenging. Whether you draw inspiration from personal stories like Sarah or global icons like The Rock, the essence remains the same: Discipline often trumps motivation. And on days it doesn't, your deep-rooted 'why' will be your guiding light. Your fitness journey is a testament to your willpower, and with the right tools and mindset, there's no stopping you. After all, as they say, "It's a slow process, but quitting won't speed it up."

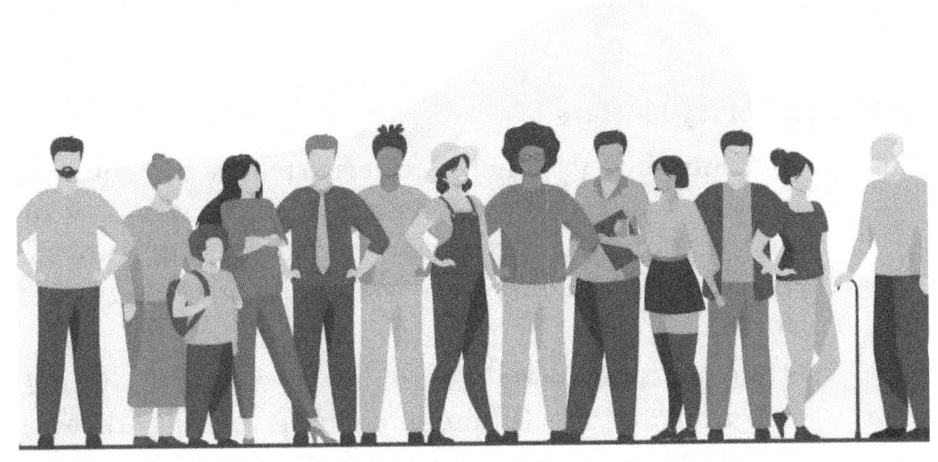

*Chapter 30:*

*The Role of Community*

*"Alone we can do so little; together we can do so much."* - Helen Keller

Imagine setting out on a journey. You have the best map, the most comfortable shoes, and a backpack filled with all you need. Yet, if the road is desolate and you're walking alone, the journey might seem daunting. Now, picture the same journey with a group of enthusiastic, supportive companions. The difference is palpable. That's the role of community in our fitness journeys.

**From Zero to Hero: Tom's Transformation**

Tom, a chubby software developer, always sat in the back during team photos. He was conscious of his weight but had accepted it as his identity. One day, a colleague invited him to a local community running group. Initially hesitant, Tom eventually decided to give it a go. Fast forward two years, Tom had not only shed the extra pounds but had also finished his first half marathon, all thanks to the unwavering support of his running community.

## Why Community Matters

1. **Accountability:** When you're part of a community, there's a sense of responsibility. Skipping a day or cheating on your diet doesn't just affect you; it affects the group. This sense of answerability can be a driving force.

2. **Shared Knowledge:** Communities are gold mines of information. Different members bring diverse experiences, tricks, tips, and strategies that can immensely benefit the group.

3. **Emotional Support:** On days when motivation runs low, having someone to share your struggles with can be comforting.

## Arnold Schwarzenegger and the Golden Age of Bodybuilding

The world knows Arnold for his acting, politics, and his impressive physique. But behind those muscles was a close-knit community of bodybuilders in the Golden Era. Training at the famous Gold's Gym in Venice, California, these individuals thrived on camaraderie. They trained together, ate together, and grew together. The supportive atmosphere played a pivotal role in shaping their careers.

## Daily Tasks and Training Program

**Daily Tasks:**

1. **Engage Actively:** Actively participate in community activities, be it online discussions or offline meetups.

2. **Share and Learn:** Don't just take; give back by sharing

your experiences, progress, and knowledge.

3. **Celebrate Together:** Celebrate not just your milestones but also those of other community members.

## 4-Week Community-Driven Fitness Program:

- **Week 1:** *Integration Phase*
  - **Day 1-3:** Join a local or online fitness community. Introduce yourself and get to know members.
  - **Day 4-7:** Attend group training sessions or participate in community challenges.

- **Week 2:** *Engagement Phase*
  - **Day 1-3:** Engage in community discussions. Share your fitness goals and progress.
  - **Day 4-7:** Collaborate with a community member for a combined workout or diet plan.

- **Week 3:** *Contribution Phase*
  - **Day 1-3:** Share a personal fitness story or write a blog post/tutorial.
  - **Day 4-7:** Organize or assist in a community event – a group run, yoga session, or diet planning workshop.

- **Week 4:** *Feedback and Growth Phase*
  - **Day 1-3:** Seek feedback on your techniques, diet, or routines.
  - **Day 4-7:** Reflect on the feedback, adjust your routines, and set goals for the next month.

## Actionable Strategies:

1. **Choose the Right Community:** Not every group might be a good fit. Ensure that the community aligns with

your goals and values.

2. **Be Consistent:** Regularly engage with the community. This consistency fosters trust and relationships.

3. **Go Beyond Digital:** If possible, attend physical meet-ups or organize one. Physical interactions often lead to stronger bonds.

### Food for Thought: Is it Only About Fitness?

While fitness communities revolve around health and wellness, they often offer more. Friendships, networking, emotional support, and sometimes even love! These communities become microcosms of society, teaching values like patience, empathy, and perseverance.

### Summary:

A fitness journey, while personal, doesn't have to be lonely. Integrating into a community can be the game-changer you were looking for. Whether it's the shared sense of purpose, collective knowledge, or the simple joy of togetherness, communities play an indispensable role in making our fitness quests fulfilling. As Tom found his stride amidst fellow runners and Arnold sculpted his legacy alongside fellow bodybuilders, may you find your tribe that pushes you towards your best self. Because at the end of the day, we all need someone to high-five after a hard workout or to tell us, "One more rep, you got this!"

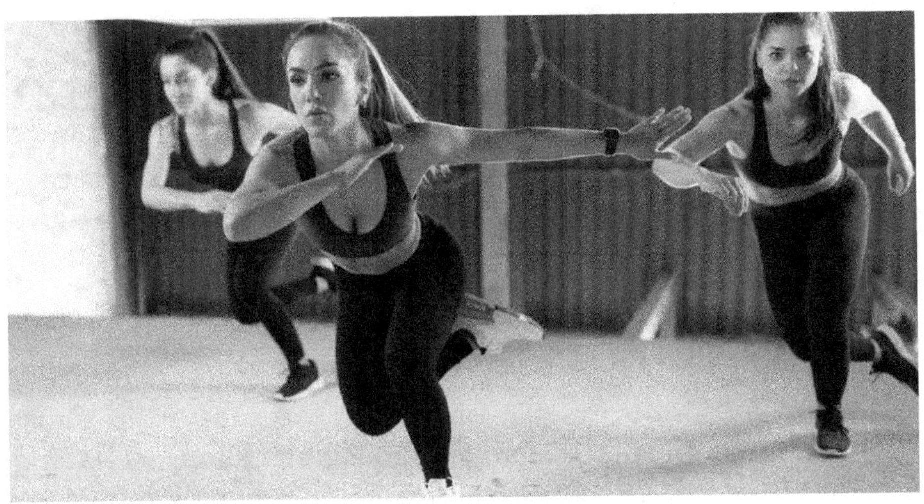

## Chapter 31:

## High-Intensity Training

*"It's not the time you spend working out; it's the intensity with which you do it. Quality over quantity!"*

A few decades ago, the buzzword 'High-Intensity Training' (HIT) might have sounded alien to many. Today, it's a staple in the world of fitness. But what makes this workout methodology so unique and effective? Let's delve deeper into HIT's universe.

### Sweating it Out with Michael

Michael, a busy corporate lawyer, barely had an hour to spare for his fitness routines. Traditional gym workouts seemed to take forever, and results were slow. Then, a colleague introduced him to HIT. In just 20 minutes, Michael felt more exhausted than he had in an hour of his usual routine. Within months, he was leaner, stronger, and more energetic, all thanks to the power of high intensity.

## What is High-Intensity Training (HIT)?

HIT involves short, intense bursts of exercise, followed by a brief rest period. These workouts can range from 15 to 30 minutes, making them perfect for those pressed for time. Yet, the catch is in the 'intensity'. During the active phase, you're expected to give it your all, pushing your body to its limit.

## The Science Behind HIT

- **Caloric Burn:** HIT can torch calories in a short time. The sheer intensity boosts metabolism, leading to a higher post-exercise caloric burn, known as the 'afterburn' or EPOC (Excess Post-exercise Oxygen Consumption).

- **Improved Cardiovascular Health:** Engaging the heart in these vigorous bursts improves cardiovascular strength and stamina.

- **Muscle Preservation:** Unlike steady-state cardio, which might burn muscle along with fat, HIT, when combined with strength exercises, can preserve lean muscle mass.

## Tabata: HIT in Action

Dr. Izumi Tabata, a Japanese researcher, introduced a form of HIT now known as the 'Tabata Protocol'. In his study, Olympic speed-skaters trained 4 times a week using a formula: 20 seconds of ultra-intense exercise followed by 10 seconds of rest, repeated 8 times. The results? Improved aerobic and anaerobic pathways, making it a dual win.

## Daily Tasks and Training Program

**Daily Tasks:**

1. **Warm-Up:** Before any HIT session, ensure a 5-10 minute warm-up to prepare your body.

2. **Stay Hydrated:** Intense workouts can lead to rapid water loss. Keep a water bottle handy.

3. **Track Progress:** Log your workouts, noting down exercises, durations, and repetitions. This helps gauge improvements.

**4-Week HIT Program:**

- **Week 1:** *Introduction*
    - **Day 1-2:** 30 seconds of high-intensity exercise (like sprinting) followed by 30 seconds rest. Repeat for 15 minutes.
    - **Day 3-5:** Incorporate bodyweight exercises (burpees, push-ups, squats). 30 seconds on, 30 seconds rest.
    - **Day 6-7:** Rest or light activity like walking.
- **Week 2:** *Upping the Intensity*
    - **Day 1-3:** Increase active phase to 40 seconds, with 20 seconds rest.
    - **Day 4-5:** Introduce weights or resistance bands.
    - **Day 6-7:** Active recovery - gentle yoga or stretching.
- **Week 3:** *Challenge Week*
    - **Day 1-2:** Tabata Protocol – 20 seconds on, 10 seconds off.
    - **Day 3-4:** HIT circuit training – choose 5 exercises, do each at high intensity for 40 seconds, 20 seconds rest in between.

- **Day 5:** Longer HIT session – 30 minutes.
    - **Day 6-7:** Rest.
  - **Week 4:** *Consolidation Phase*
    - **Day 1-5:** Mix and match from the routines of the past three weeks.
    - **Day 6-7:** Rest and rejuvenation.

## Actionable Strategies:

1. **Listen to Your Body:** HIT is demanding. If you ever feel it's too much, scale back.

2. **Diversity is Key:** Ensure a mix of cardio and strength exercises for holistic fitness.

3. **Seek Expert Advice:** Before starting any HIT program, especially if you have medical conditions, consult a fitness professional.

## Food for Thought: The 'Intensity' of Life

Isn't life a bit like HIT? We have moments of sheer intensity, followed by periods of rest and recovery. Just as our muscles grow stronger with each HIT session, our character gets fortified with life's challenges. The key lies in embracing the intensity, pushing through, and allowing adequate recovery.

## Summary:

High-Intensity Training, though grueling, is a testament to the saying, "What doesn't kill you makes you stronger." In a world where 'time' is a luxury, HIT stands as a beacon for fitness enthusiasts. While Michael found his fitness elixir in the form of HIT, each one of us can find our rhythm. Whether you're an athlete or someone just starting, the world of HIT has something for everyone. Just remember, as with life, it's not about how long you work but how effectively you do it.

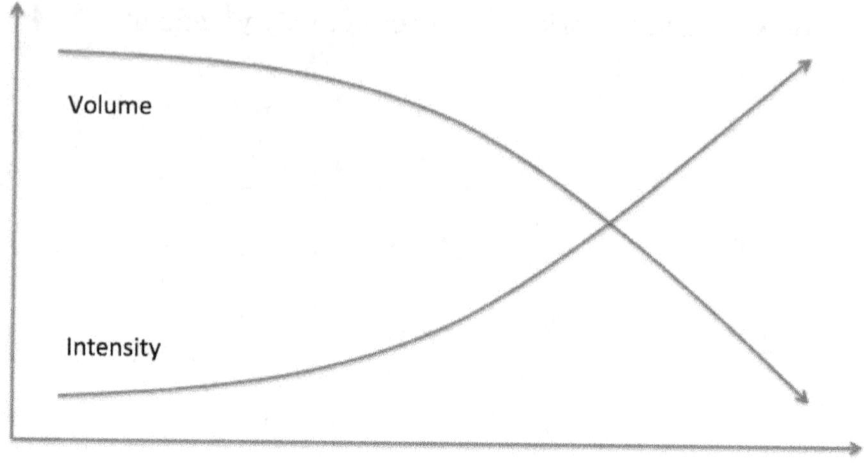


## Chapter 32:

## Periodization: Planning for Long-term Success

*"A goal without a plan is just a wish." - Antoine de Saint-Exupéry*

While many of us start our fitness journey with abundant enthusiasm, it's the planning and structure that determine our success. Enter the world of 'Periodization', the science-backed strategy that elite athletes and professionals swear by.

**Chasing Olympic Gold:** The Matthew Story

In the early 2000s, Matthew, a young swimmer, had just one dream: to win an Olympic gold. Although he trained rigorously every day, his performance was a roller coaster. It was only when his coach introduced periodized training that Matthew started to see consistent improvements. Not only did he bag the gold in 2008, but he also set a new world record!

**Unraveling Periodization**

Periodization is a systematic approach to training that involves breaking down the annual training schedule into manageable phases or cycles. Each phase focuses on specific fitness development aspects, ensuring the athlete peaks at the right time, say, during a competition.

## The Science Behind Periodization

- **Avoiding Plateaus:** Constantly varying your training stimulus ensures that the body doesn't adapt to one type of training, avoiding performance stagnation.

- **Reducing Injury Risks:** By cycling between high-intensity training and low-intensity recovery periods, periodization reduces overuse injuries.

- **Optimal Performance:** Periodization plans for peak performance. By methodically increasing intensity and volume, the athlete reaches their top form right when it matters.

## The Different Cycles of Periodization

1. **Macrocycle:** Typically, this refers to the annual plan, though it can span longer.

2. **Mesocycle:** This is a phase within the macrocycle, typically lasting 4-6 weeks, focusing on a particular fitness attribute.

3. **Microcycle:** A week within a mesocycle, detailing the specific workouts and their objectives.

## Daily Tasks and Training Program

## Daily Tasks:

1. **Log Your Training:** Keep a detailed journal of your

exercises, sets, reps, and feelings.

2. **Listen to Your Body**: Make adjustments based on how you feel. Tired? It might be time for a deload week.

3. **Nutrition & Sleep**: Ensure adequate nutrient intake and sleep as they play pivotal roles in recovery.

**Sample 12-Week Periodized Program:**

- **Week 1-4**: Endurance Phase (Mesocycle 1)
    - **Focus:** Building a base, improving cardiovascular endurance.
    - **Daily:** 30-60 minutes of low to moderate-intensity cardio.
    - **Strength Training:** 3 days a week, 2-3 sets of 12-15 reps, lighter weights.
- **Week 5-8**: Strength Phase (Mesocycle 2)
    - **Focus:** Developing muscle strength.
    - **Strength Training**: 4 days a week, 3-4 sets of 6-8 reps, heavier weights.
    - **Daily:** Incorporate interval training for cardio, 20-30 minutes.
- **Week 9-11**: Power Phase (Mesocycle 3)
    - **Focus:** Enhancing muscle power.
    - **Strength Training:** 3 days a week, 3-4 sets of 3-5 reps, using even heavier weights or explosive movements like plyometrics.
    - **Daily:** Mix steady-state cardio with high-intensity bursts.
- **Week 12**: Tapering and Recovery
    - Reduce training intensity and volume to recover and prepare for peak performance.

**Actionable Strategies:**

1. **Seek Expert Guidance:** If you're new to periodization, consider hiring a trainer or coach to guide you.

2. **Be Flexible:** Periodization is a roadmap, not a strict rulebook. Adjust based on needs and unforeseen challenges.

3. **Include Mental Training:** Especially if you're prepping for a competition, include visualization and relaxation techniques in your mesocycles.

**Food for Thought:** The Rhythms of Life

Life, like training, has its seasons. There are times of growth, moments of reflection, and periods of recovery. Periodization isn't just a training principle; it mirrors life's rhythm. The key lies in recognizing which 'season' we are in and adapting accordingly.

**Summary:**

Periodization is the art and science of training organization. It's a testament to the saying, "Failing to plan is planning to fail." This structured approach offers a roadmap to your fitness goals, be it winning a gold medal or just improving overall health. It teaches us to respect our body's rhythm, to push, to pull back, and to peak at the right moment. In life and in fitness, it's all about timing. Remember, it's not always about how hard you train, but how smartly you do it.

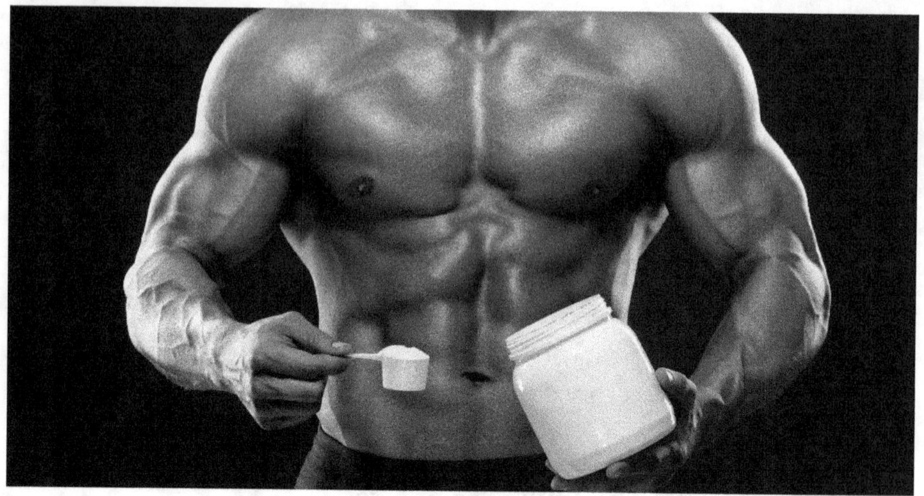

## Chapter 33:

## Advanced Nutrition for Athletes

*"Let food be thy medicine, and medicine be thy food." – Hippocrates*

The role of nutrition transcends mere sustenance; for athletes, it's the cornerstone of peak performance. As the stakes heighten and milliseconds become the difference between gold and silver, advanced nutrition becomes the unsung hero of athletic success.

**Eating Gold:** The Serena Williams Transformation

In the realm of tennis, few names shine as brightly as Serena Williams. But did you know that at the peak of her career, Serena made a drastic dietary shift? Aiming to optimize her performance and manage some health concerns, she embraced a plant-based diet. The result? A revitalized energy on the court and a continued dominance in her sport. Her story underscores the immense impact of tailored nutrition.

**Beyond Basic Macros:** The World of Advanced Nutrition

While understanding macronutrients (carbs, fats, proteins) is essential, athletes often delve deeper into:

1. **Micronutrients:** Vital vitamins and minerals that optimize metabolic pathways, muscle function, and bone health.

2. **Hydration:** A game-changer in stamina, recovery, and cognitive function.

3. **Nutrient Timing:** Aligning intake to maximize recovery and performance.

4. **Supplementation:** Bridging nutritional gaps or elevating performance.

## The Science of Fueling Performance

- **Carbohydrates:** The primary energy source during high-intensity activities. The glycogen stores in our muscles stem from carbs and offer the immediate energy surge needed in sprints or heavy lifts.

- **Proteins:** Essential for muscle repair and growth. A continuous supply helps in speedy recovery and muscle development.

- **Fats:** They play a role during prolonged, lower-intensity exercises, acting as a vast energy reserve.

## Daily Tasks and Training Program

**Daily Tasks:**

1. **Monitor Intake:** Track what you eat. Apps like MyFitnessPal can help.

2. **Stay Hydrated:** Aim for at least 3 liters daily, more if you're in intense training.

3. **Pre-and Post-Workout Nutrition:** Never neglect the crucial meals before and after training.

## Sample Nutrition Program for Endurance Athletes:

### Breakfast:

- Oatmeal with blueberries, chia seeds, and almond milk.
- Scrambled tofu with spinach and tomatoes.

### Lunch:

- Quinoa salad with roasted veggies, avocado, and a lemon-tahini dressing.
- Lentil soup with whole-grain bread.

### Pre-workout Snack:

- Banana and almond butter.
- A hydration drink with electrolytes.

### Post-workout:

- Plant-based protein shake with almond milk.
- Sweet potato with steamed broccoli.

### Dinner:

- Grilled tempeh with asparagus and brown rice.
- Mixed fruit bowl.

## Actionable Strategies:

1. **Consult a Sports Nutritionist:** Tailor your diet to your specific needs.

2. **Diversify Your Diet:** Ensure you're getting a range of nutrients by eating a colorful array of foods.

3. **Read Up on Supplements:** Not all supplements are created equal. Research and choose high-quality

options that match your goals.

**Food for Thought:** Nutrition as an Extension of Training

It's easy to dissociate nutrition from training, viewing them as two distinct entities. However, think of nutrition as an extension of your training — the two are symbiotic. The effort you exert in the gym, on the track, or in the pool is deeply intertwined with the fuel you provide your body.

**Summary:**

Advanced nutrition for athletes is about precision, understanding that every morsel you consume can influence your performance. It's not merely about quantity but the quality and timing of nutrients. Whether you're an aspiring athlete or a seasoned one, taking a leaf out of Serena's book — recognizing and adapting to the unique nutritional demands of your body — can set you on a path to unprecedented success. After all, true athletic prowess is not just built in the training grounds, but also in the kitchen.

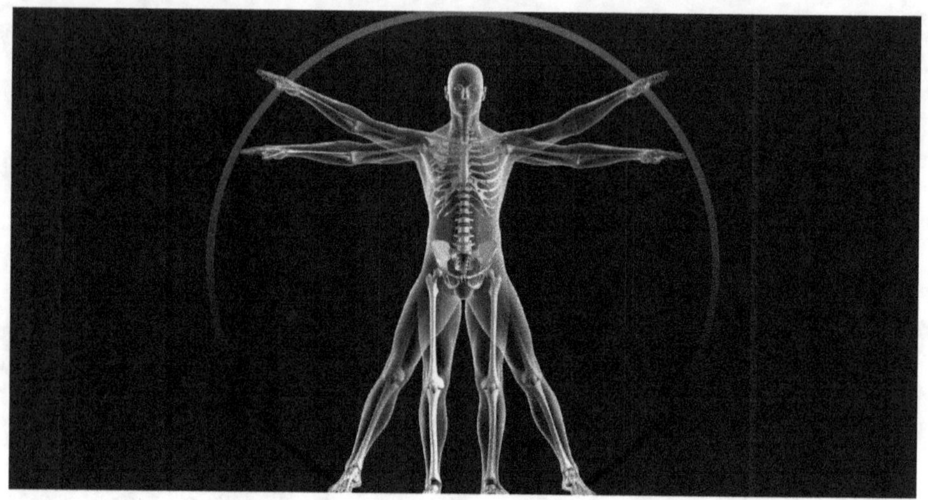

## Chapter 34:

## Biohacking Your Fitness

*"Your body is your most priceless possession, so go take care of it." – Jack LaLanne*

Biohacking might sound like something out of a sci-fi movie, but it's become the buzzword in fitness circles. Simply put, biohacking is the pursuit of optimizing one's physiology through the integration of technology, nutrition, and other modalities.

**The Dave Asprey Transformation:** From Overweight to Bulletproof

If you've sipped on a creamy cup of Bulletproof coffee, you've tasted the genius of Dave Asprey. But Dave wasn't always the picture of health. Struggling with obesity and cognitive dysfunction, he embarked on a journey that led him to spend over $300,000 on testing and tweaking his biology. Through countless experiments and self-reflection, Dave not only shed weight but also honed his mental acuity. His story epitomizes biohacking's potential when wielded correctly.

## What is Biohacking, Exactly?

Biohacking is the intersection of biology and the hacker ethos. It's about understanding and modifying our internal and external environments so we can "upgrade" our bodies and minds.

## Types of Biohacking:

1. **Nutrigenomics:** How food impacts our genes and subsequently our health.

2. **Digital Detoxing:** Reducing electronic use to lower stress and improve sleep.

3. **Wearable Tech:** Devices that track everything from sleep, heart rate, to blood oxygen levels.

4. **Cryotherapy & Sauna Sessions:** Leveraging temperature for recovery and performance.

## Daily Tasks and Training Program

### Daily Tasks:

1. **Track Sleep:** Use wearable tech to ensure 7-9 hours of quality rest.

2. **Mindful Eating:** Reflect on your food choices and how they make you feel.

3. **Digital Downtime:** Dedicate an hour before bed without screens.

## Sample Biohacking Training Program:

### Monday:

- Morning: Meditation with a brainwave entrainment tool.

- Workout: High-Intensity Interval Training (HIIT).
- Evening: Cryotherapy session.

## Tuesday:

- Morning: Fast until noon to tap into intermittent fasting benefits.
- Workout: Strength training.
- Evening: Infrared sauna session.

## Wednesday:

- Morning: Bulletproof coffee to fuel the brain and body.
- Workout: Active recovery (light walk, stretching).
- Evening: Deep sleep tracking with a wearable device.

Repeat a similar structure for the rest of the week, incorporating various biohacking tools and strategies.

## Actionable Strategies:

1. **Educate Yourself:** Read up on the latest biohacking research and trends.
2. **Start Small:** Incorporate one biohacking technique and then expand.
3. **Consult Professionals:** Seek guidance from those knowledgeable in specific biohacking areas.

## Food for Thought: Nature's Biohack

While technology and modern strategies play a huge role in biohacking, it's essential to remember that nature offers its own biohacks. A sunset walk, grounding (bare feet on earth), or listening to the natural rhythm of ocean waves can optimize our well-being in profound ways.

## Summary:

Biohacking is an exciting frontier in the fitness and health domain. It offers tools and techniques that can catalyze our journey towards optimal health. But as Dave Asprey's story suggests, it's a personalized endeavor. What works wonders for one might not for another. The key is to understand, experiment, and find what's uniquely beneficial for your body and mind. With the right information and a touch of curiosity, you can leverage biohacking to propel yourself into a realm of enhanced health and performance. As always, blending the old with the new—nature with technology—can often yield the most harmonious results.

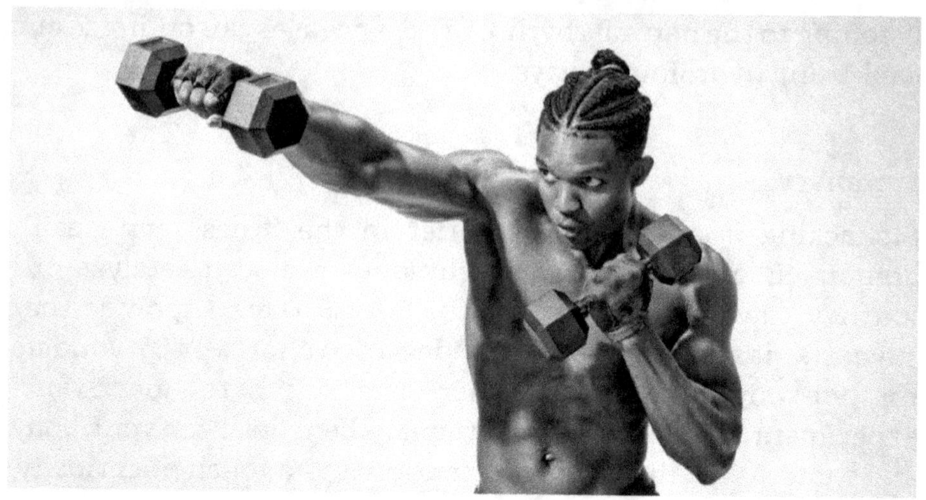

*Chapter 35:*

*Sport-Specific Training*

*"Don't practice until you get it right. Practice until you can't get it wrong." – Unknown*

Every sport, from basketball to ballet, requires a unique set of physical and mental skills. Whether you're aiming for the Olympics, the local league, or personal mastery, sport-specific training can help you hone the exact abilities you need. It's not about generic fitness; it's about becoming the best at *your* game.

## Michael Jordan: From Court to Diamond and Back Again

Many remember Michael Jordan for his basketball prowess, but in 1994, he made a shocking switch to baseball. Though an incredible athlete, Jordan initially struggled in this new domain. It wasn't until he tailored his training specifically for baseball's demands that he began to show promise. This venture was short-lived, but upon his return to basketball, Jordan's diversified training helped him add new dimensions to his game. His story drives home the message: different sports require different training.

## Why Generic Workouts Won't Cut It

Imagine training like a marathon runner when your sport is weightlifting. You'd be well-conditioned cardiovascularly but lacking in raw strength. Each sport has distinct physical demands, and your training should reflect that. Sport-specific training targets the muscles, movements, and metabolic pathways most utilized in your chosen activity.

## Elements of Sport-Specific Training:

1. **Movement Patterns:** Mimic the actual movements you'll do in your sport.

2. **Energy Systems:** Train the specific metabolic pathways predominantly used in your sport.

3. **Skill Development:** Beyond physical fitness, sports require technical mastery.

## Daily Tasks and Training Program

### Daily Tasks:

1. **Movement Drills:** Dedicate time each day to mimic specific motions of your sport.

2. **Mindset Training:** Visualize successful game scenarios or performances.

3. **Recovery:** Prioritize rest and techniques that help your body recover.

## Sample Training Program for a Tennis Player:

### Monday:

- Morning: Agility ladder drills for footwork.
- Workout: Upper body strength training focused on overhead pressing (serving motion).
- Evening: Stretching and foam rolling, emphasizing the shoulders and hips.

**Tuesday:**

- Morning: Serve practice with focus on technique.
- Workout: Cardio interval training mimicking match point scenarios.
- Evening: Meditation and visualization of match-winning plays.

**Wednesday:**

- Morning: Return drills with a partner.
- Workout: Lower body strength training with an emphasis on lunges and lateral movements.
- Evening: Epsom salt bath for muscle recovery.

This structure is then modified for the rest of the week to encompass all aspects of tennis.

**Actionable Strategies:**

1. **Seek Expertise:** Work with a coach who has experience in your sport.
2. **Analyze Top Players:** Study the greats in your sport. Break down their techniques and integrate their methods.
3. **Test and Reassess:** Regularly check your progress. Modify your regimen based on your evolving

strengths and weaknesses.

## Food for Thought: The Mental Edge

While physical training is paramount, sports often require strategic thinking and mental fortitude. The tennis player Serena Williams, for instance, is not just powerful but also a tactical genius on the court. To truly excel, ensure your training regime enhances both your body and your mind.

## Summary:

Sport-specific training is the laser-focused approach to becoming your best athletic self. By tailoring your workouts to the exact demands of your sport, you set the stage for peak performance. Remember Michael Jordan's venture into baseball: raw athleticism isn't always enough. It's the fusion of targeted physical training and mental mastery that creates a champion. Whatever your sport, train with purpose, intention, and a keen eye on the nuances of your game. The results will speak for themselves.

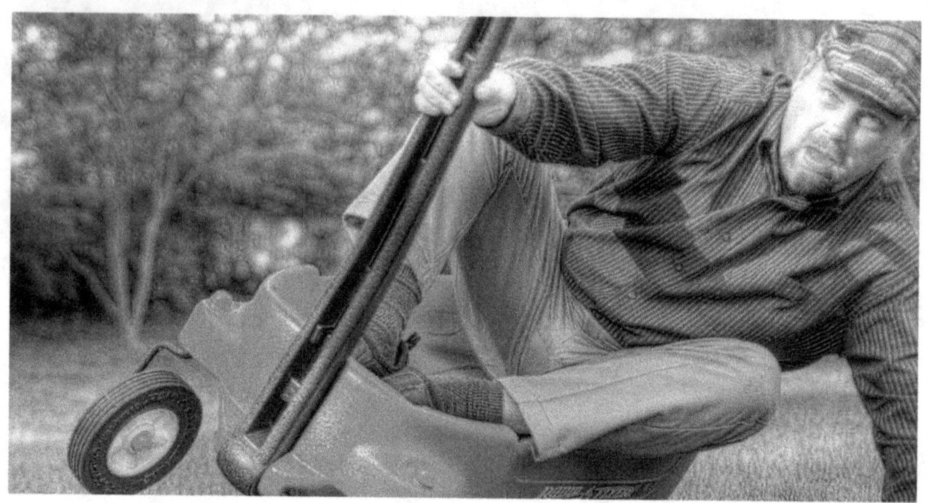

## Chapter 36:

## What to Do When You
## Fall Off the Wagon

*"Success is not final, failure is not fatal: It is the courage to continue that counts." – Winston Churchill*

We've all been there. One day you're diligently following your fitness regimen, and the next thing you know, life happens. Maybe you indulged a bit too much on vacation, got swamped at work, or faced a personal crisis. No matter the reason, the wagon has been departed, and you feel like you're back at square one.

The truth? Everyone stumbles. The difference between those who succeed and those who don't lies in their response to setbacks.

### Dwayne "The Rock" Johnson: From Rock Bottom to Rock Solid

Few embody resilience like Dwayne Johnson. Before gracing Hollywood screens or wrestling rings, Johnson had dreams of football stardom. Yet, injuries derailed his career, leading him into a depression, and he found himself with just $7 in his pocket. Instead of being consumed by his setbacks, he chose to learn, evolve, and relentlessly pursue a new path. Fitness became a cornerstone of his resurgence, and he used it as a tool to rebuild himself mentally and physically. The lesson? Falling down isn't the end—it's the opportunity for a new beginning.

## Understanding the Setback

Before making a triumphant return to your fitness journey, it's crucial to understand why you veered off course.

Common Reasons for Falling Off:

1. **Overambitious Goals:** Aiming too high, too soon can lead to burnout.
2. **Lack of Enjoyment:** If you don't love your workout, it's hard to stick to it.
3. **Life Changes:** From illness to new job responsibilities, life's unpredictability can disrupt routines.

**Daily Tasks and Training Program:** Getting Back on Track

## Daily Tasks:

1. **Reflection:** Spend 10 minutes journaling about what caused the setback.
2. **Affirmations:** Repeat positive mantras emphasizing resilience and self-love.
3. **Small Actions:** Do one thing for your fitness, even if it's just a 10-minute walk.

## 4-Week Reboot Program:

**Week 1:** Gentle Restart

- **Monday to Sunday:** 20-minute walks daily, focusing on breathing and enjoying the movement.

**Week 2:** Introducing Structure

- **Monday/Wednesday/Friday:** 30-minute light cardio (jogging, cycling).
- **Tuesday/Thursday:** Basic bodyweight exercises - push-ups, squats, and lunges.

**Week 3:** Upping the Intensity

- **Monday/Wednesday/Friday:** Cardio intervals—1 minute running, 1-minute walking for 30 minutes.
- **Tuesday/Thursday:** Bodyweight strength training, adding in planks and step-ups.

**Week 4:** Diversify and Challenge

- **Monday:** Cardio, 40 minutes with increased intensity.
- **Tuesday:** Strength training with light weights.
- **Wednesday:** Flexibility—Yoga or Pilates.
- **Thursday:** Cardio intervals with uphill variations.
- **Friday:** Full-body strength training.
- **Weekend:** Rest and light recreational activities like hiking or swimming.

**Actionable Strategies:**

1. **Reset Your Goals:** Aim for realistic, short-term milestones.

2. **Seek Support:** Join a fitness group, hire a coach, or find a workout buddy.

3. **Celebrate Small Wins:** Every time you achieve even a minor goal, reward yourself (non-food rewards are preferable).

**Food for Thought:** The Bigger Picture

Fitness is a journey, not a destination. In the grand scheme of things, a setback is just a tiny fraction of your story. In fact, many find that after a hiatus, they return with renewed vigor, perspective, and appreciation for their health. Instead of punishing yourself, use this as an opportunity to cultivate resilience, adaptability, and self-compassion.

**Summary:**

Setbacks are an inevitable part of the fitness journey, but they're not the end. Remember Dwayne Johnson's story—from near despair to global stardom, with fitness playing a pivotal role in his resurgence. Whether you've fallen off the wagon for a week, a month, or a year, what matters most is your determination to climb back on. Approach your comeback with understanding, realistic goals, and the belief that every setback is a setup for a greater comeback. Fitness isn't about being perfect—it's about being persistent. Embrace the ebb and flow, and always strive to be the best version of yourself.

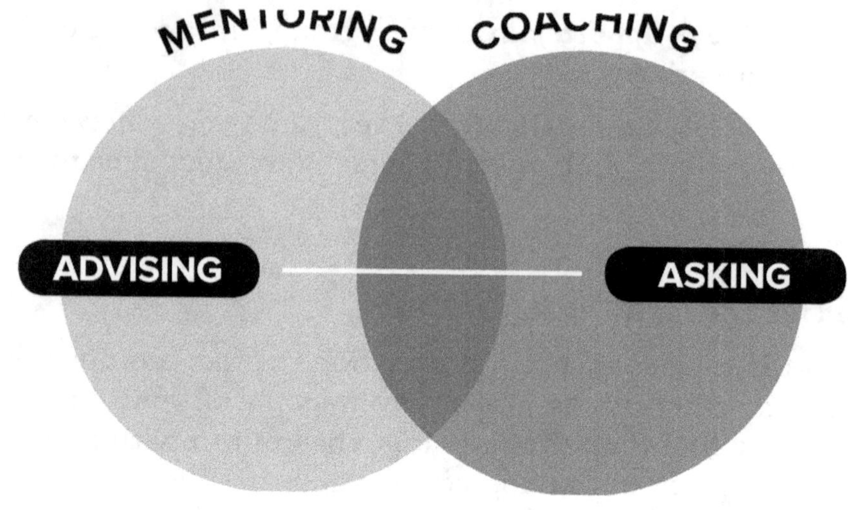


## Chapter 37:

## The Role of Coaching and Mentorship

*"I am not a teacher, but an awakener." – Robert Frost*

In every hero's journey, there's a mentor who guides, supports, and elevates. Think of Luke Skywalker and Yoda, Harry Potter and Dumbledore, or even Rocky Balboa and Mickey Goldmill. Behind many success stories, especially in the world of fitness, there's often a coach or mentor playing a pivotal role.

**Serena Williams and Patrick Mouratoglou:** A Partnership Beyond the Court

When Serena Williams, one of the greatest tennis players of all time, faced a slump in her career in 2012, she sought the guidance of French coach Patrick Mouratoglou. While already a champion, Serena understood the need for a fresh perspective to elevate her game further. Under Patrick's mentorship, Serena won 10 of her 23 Grand Slam singles titles. Their relationship transcended typical player-coach dynamics—it was a partnership founded on trust, mutual respect, and shared ambition.

## Why Coaching and Mentorship Matter

### 1. Expertise and Experience:

A seasoned coach provides tried-and-true strategies, helping you avoid common pitfalls and achieve results more efficiently.

### 2. Accountability:

Having someone to answer to can be the difference between hitting the snooze button and hitting the gym.

### 3. Personalized Feedback:

While there's a wealth of fitness information available, a coach can tailor advice specifically for you, considering your strengths, weaknesses, and goals.

### 4. Emotional Support:

The fitness journey has its highs and lows. A coach or mentor serves as a pillar of support, helping you navigate challenges with resilience.

**Daily Tasks and Training Program:** Leveraging Coaching for Optimal Growth

**Daily Tasks:**

1. **Check-in:** Begin your day with a brief conversation with your coach or mentor, discussing your goals for

the day and any potential challenges.

2. **Training Journal:** Document your workouts, noting how you felt, what went well, and areas of struggle. Share this with your coach for feedback.

3. **Reflection:** End your day by reflecting on your progress, lessons learned, and how your coach's guidance influenced your decisions.

**4-Week Growth-Driven Program with a Coach:**

**Week 1:** Assessment and Foundation Building

- **Daily:** Engage in baseline tests to gauge your fitness level.

- **Feedback Sessions:** Post-assessment, discuss your goals, strengths, and areas of improvement with your coach.

**Week 2:** Targeted Skill Development

- **Monday to Friday:** Focus on one key area each day (e.g., strength, endurance, flexibility, balance, and agility).

- **Feedback Sessions:** Daily check-ins to discuss progress, challenges, and adjustments.

**Week 3:** Integration and Challenge

- **Monday/Wednesday/Friday:** Full-body workouts integrating the week 2 focus areas.

- **Tuesday/Thursday:** Recovery and technique refinement sessions.

- **Feedback Sessions:** Bi-weekly deep dives into progress, ensuring proper form and addressing any pain points.

**Week 4:** Mastery and Forward Planning

- **Daily:** Advanced workouts tailored to your goals, pushing your limits.
- **Feedback Sessions:** Reflect on the month's progress, celebrating successes, and planning the next phase of your fitness journey.

**Actionable Strategies:**

1. **Choose Wisely:** Not all coaches are created equal. Ensure your chosen coach aligns with your goals, values, and learning style.
2. **Be Open and Honest:** The more transparent you are about your challenges, fears, and aspirations, the better equipped your coach will be to guide you.
3. **Commit Fully:** Like any relationship, the coach-mentee dynamic thrives on commitment. Fully invest in the process, trust your coach, and be open to feedback.

**Food for Thought:** Beyond the Physical

A coach does more than guide your physical journey—they often play a pivotal role in mental growth. The confidence gained from conquering a challenging workout, the discipline learned from consistent training, or the resilience built from bouncing back after setbacks—these lessons often parallel life's broader challenges. In essence, a good coach doesn't just train your body; they empower your spirit.

**Summary:**

In the realm of fitness, as in many aspects of life, guidance from someone more experienced can be invaluable. Whether you're a newbie seeking direction or a seasoned athlete aiming for new heights, the role of coaching and mentorship can't be overstated. Remember the partnership between Serena Williams and Patrick Mouratoglou—it wasn't just about perfecting a serve or forehand. It was about shared ambition, mutual growth, and a commitment to excellence. As you embark or continue on your fitness journey, consider seeking a mentor or coach. In doing so, you're not just investing in your physical well-being but also nurturing your growth as a holistic individual.

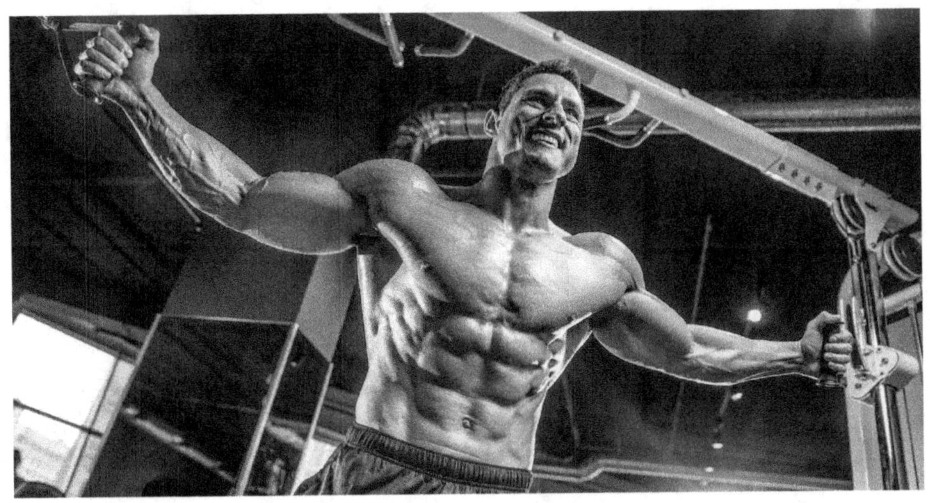

## Chapter 38:

## Review and Adjust: Your Evolving Fitness Plan

*"It is not the strongest of the species that survives, nor the most intelligent that survives. It is the one that is the most adaptable to change." – Charles Darwin*

No path is a straight line, and your fitness journey won't be either. As we progress, our bodies adapt, goals evolve, and external factors (like work or personal commitments) change. Therefore, consistently reviewing and adjusting your fitness plan is vital to ensure sustained progress and motivation.

### Chris Hemsworth: A Shape-shifting Marvel

From the godly physique of Thor to the lean form of a sailor stranded at sea in "In the Heart of the Sea," Chris Hemsworth's body transformations have been nothing short of remarkable. The secret? Constantly evolving training regimes and dietary plans tailored to specific roles. Hemsworth and his trainer review and adjust depending on the actor's upcoming roles and current physical condition. Their adaptability showcases the importance of never settling and always striving for the next goal.

## Why Reviewing and Adjusting is Imperative

### 1. Preventing Plateaus:

The body is an incredible adaptive machine. Do the same workout repeatedly, and it will adapt, resulting in slowed progress or even stagnation.

### 2. Avoiding Overuse Injuries:

Varying workouts can prevent the repetitive strain on specific muscles or joints, reducing injury risk.

### 3. Keeping Things Fresh and Motivating:

Changing up your routine can reignite your passion and motivation for fitness, preventing boredom or burnout.

**Daily Tasks and Training Program:** The Art of Adaptability

**Daily Tasks:**

1. **Monitor Feedback:** How does your body feel post-workout? Energetic, drained, or somewhere in between? Jot down daily feedback.
2. **Stay Updated:** Dedicate 10 minutes daily to read or watch something new related to fitness. Staying informed can offer new techniques or insights to integrate.
3. **Mindful Reflection:** Before bed, reflect on your

emotional response to your workout. Did you enjoy it? Why or why not?

**4-Week Adaptive Program:**

**Week 1:** Baseline Week

- **Daily:** Perform your current routine.
- **Feedback Sessions:** Note how each session feels. Are certain exercises too easy or too challenging?

**Week 2:** Variation Exploration

- **Monday to Friday:** Introduce one new exercise or modify an existing one daily.
- **Feedback Sessions:** Observe how these changes affect your energy, mood, and motivation.

**Week 3:** Integration

- **Daily:** Based on feedback from week 2, integrate the most effective changes into your routine.
- **Feedback Sessions:** Is this new routine more effective than the baseline week?

**Week 4:** Fine-tuning and Forward Planning

- **Daily:** Continue with the integrated routine, making any minor adjustments as needed.
- **Feedback Session:** Reflect on the month's progress and how the changes impacted your fitness journey. Plan the next phase with these insights in mind.

## Actionable Strategies:

1. **Seek External Feedback:** Sometimes, an external perspective can offer insights you might overlook. Consider working with a trainer periodically or join group classes for fresh ideas.

2. **Listen to Your Body:** Your body offers constant feedback. Feeling persistent aches or lack of energy might indicate the need for change.

3. **Set Short-term Milestones:** While long-term goals provide direction, short-term milestones can offer points for regular review.

**Food for Thought:** The Power of Iteration

In the tech world, there's a concept called "iteration." It's about making consistent, incremental changes to software based on feedback, leading to continuous improvement. This concept is equally applicable to fitness. By viewing your fitness plan as an "iterative" process, where regular feedback leads to small, meaningful adjustments, you create a dynamic, responsive, and effective strategy tailored to your ever-evolving needs.

**Summary:**

Sticking religiously to one routine might feel comforting, but as the inspiring shifts in Chris Hemsworth's training showcase, evolution is key. An effective fitness plan is dynamic, not static. It evolves in response to feedback, both internal (from your body and mind) and external (from trainers, peers, or new research). Embrace change, welcome adaptability, and let this iterative approach guide you towards a healthier, stronger version of yourself. Fitness, after all, is not just a destination but a journey of constant growth, learning, and transformation.

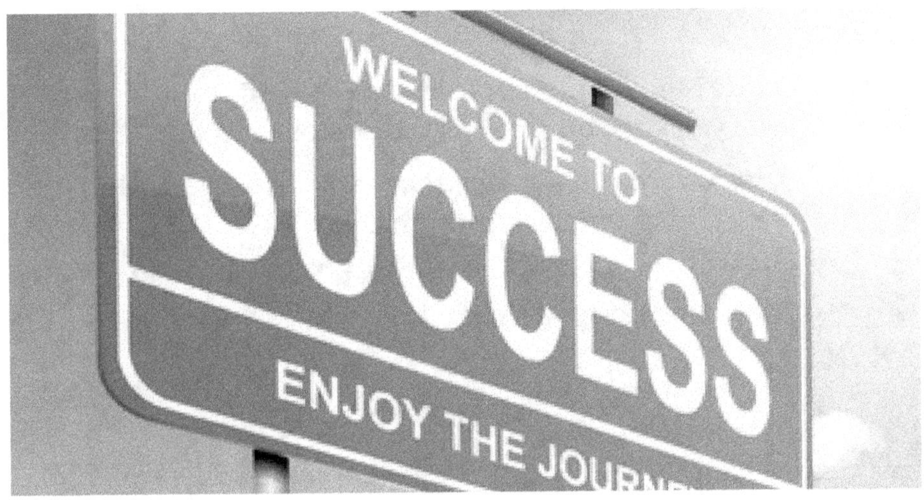


## Chapter 39:

## Case Studies: Real-life Success Stories

*"Success usually comes to those who are too busy to be looking for it."*
– Henry David Thoreau

The journey to fitness is unique for every individual. While we've delved into methods, strategies, and tools, nothing beats real-life tales of triumph to inspire and educate. In this chapter, we're pulling back the curtain on a few individuals whose fitness stories have motivated countless others.

### Sarah: The Working Mom

Sarah, a 35-year-old mother of two, juggled a demanding job, family responsibilities, and her health. At 220 lbs, she felt sluggish and was plagued by persistent backaches. Sarah decided to reclaim her health, aiming not for a "beach body," but to be an active, energetic mom.

**Strategy:**

- **Time Management:** Sarah woke up 30 minutes earlier every day to squeeze in a quick workout.
- **Diet Overhaul:** Replaced processed snacks with fruits, vegetables, and lean proteins.
- **Family Involvement:** Weekend family hikes, bike rides, and active games.

**Result:**

In a year, Sarah lost 60 lbs, but more importantly, she gained boundless energy and set a healthy example for her children.

## Tom: The Retiree Rediscovery

Tom, a 65-year-old retiree, had let himself go. After retiring, he took to a sedentary life, leading to weight gain and a decline in mental health. A wake-up call came when he struggled to play with his grandkids.

**Strategy:**

- **Joining a Senior Fitness Class:** This provided both exercise and social interaction.
- **Mindful Eating:** Tom began to understand and respect his hunger cues.
- **Daily Walks:** Tom committed to a daily 30-minute walk, rain or shine.

**Result:**

Tom not only lost 40 lbs in 8 months but rediscovered the joys of active living and formed new friendships in his fitness class.

**Jake Gyllenhaal:** From Actor to Boxer

While many know Jake Gyllenhaal for his superb acting, few are aware of his drastic physical transformation for the movie "Southpaw". Playing a boxer required him to be in peak physical condition.

**Strategy:**

- **Intensive Training:** Two workouts a day, seven days a week.
- **Boxing:** Three hours of boxing in the morning.
- **Cardio & Strength Training:** Running, jump rope, and circuit training in the evening.
- **Diet:** High protein, low carbs, and lots of water.

**Result:**

Jake not only looked the part but was able to perform his own boxing scenes, showcasing the effectiveness of his rigorous regime.

**Daily Tasks and Training Program:**

**For Sarah:**

- **Daily:** Early morning workouts focused on high-intensity interval training (HIIT).
- **Weekly:** Incorporate strength training exercises three times a week.
- **Monthly:** Family hikes or any activity involving kids.

**For Tom:**

- **Daily:** Morning walks and evening stretches.
- **Weekly:** Attend senior fitness classes thrice a week.

- **Monthly:** Try a new physical activity, from dancing to swimming.

**For Jake:**

- **Daily:** Morning boxing sessions and evening cardio and strength training.
- **Weekly:** Increase weight or resistance to challenge muscles.
- **Monthly:** Spar with professional boxers to improve skills.

**Actionable Strategies:**

1. **Find Your "Why":** Sarah wanted to be there for her kids, Tom wanted active grandparenting, and Jake had a role to nail. What's your reason?
2. **Consistency Over Intensity:** All three stuck to their routines consistently. You don't need to train like Jake – even daily walks like Tom can make a difference.
3. **Seek Support:** A supportive environment, whether family, fitness classes, or professional trainers, can make the journey enjoyable and sustainable.

**Food for Thought:** Beyond the Scale

While all our case studies experienced weight loss, their true successes lay in non-scale victories. Sarah could play with her kids without getting winded; Tom could relish his retirement actively, and Jake achieved professional accolades for a physically demanding role. The journey to fitness isn't about the numbers on a scale but about the quality of life you gain.

**Summary:**

Real-life success stories, be they of everyday heroes like Sarah and Tom or celebrities like Jake Gyllenhaal, show us the transformative power of fitness. Their strategies, while diverse, center on finding personal motivation, being consistent, and enjoying the process. Let their stories inspire you to carve your own path, remembering always to measure success not just by physical changes but by the enhanced quality of life. Fitness is personal, but success stories like these remind us that transformation is possible for everyone.

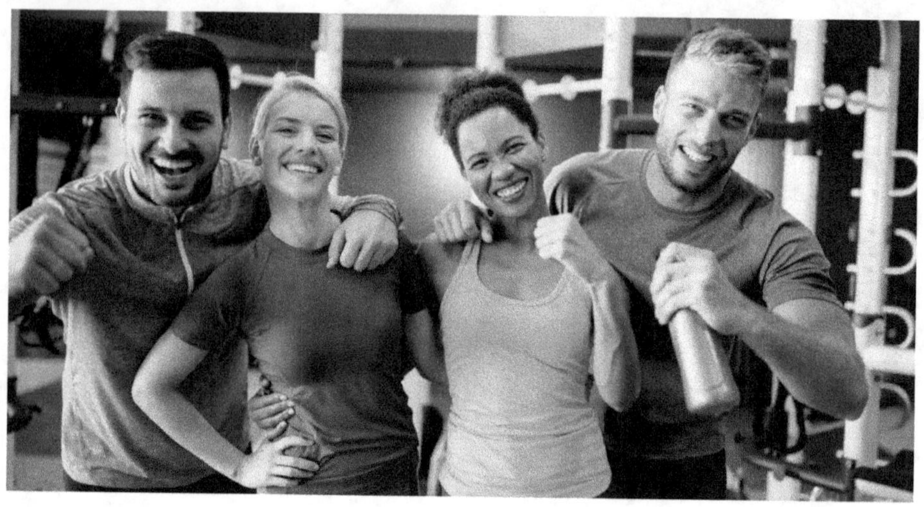

## *Chapter 40:*

## *Conclusion: Your Future in Fitness*

*"Fitness is not about being better than someone else, it's about being better than you used to be."* – Khloe Kardashian

The road to fitness isn't a sprint; it's a marathon. As we draw this book to a close, remember that your fitness journey is just beginning. Through these chapters, we've navigated the multi-faceted dimensions of fitness, from mental health to advanced nutrition, and from sport-specific training to dealing with setbacks. As you take your steps forward, it's essential to reflect, plan, and, most importantly, believe.

**Looking Back to Look Forward**

**Liam's Tale**

Liam, a middle-aged software engineer, found himself overweight and battling a host of health issues. At 45, he decided to pivot his sedentary life. He started with slow walks around his block, which led to jogging, then running. Today, Liam is a celebrated local marathon runner, proving that age is just a number.

This anecdote exemplifies that it's never too late to start. And while the finish line is fulfilling, the journey there is equally rewarding. Your path, like Liam's, will be filled with personal victories, challenges, and moments of introspection. But remember, every step counts.

**Daily Tasks and Training Program**

**The Future Fitness Checklist:**

1. **Journaling:** Spend 5 minutes daily reflecting on your fitness achievements, challenges, and feelings. It serves as a barometer for your progress.

2. **Setting Micro-Goals:** Each week, pinpoint a minor goal to achieve. It could be adding 5 minutes to your workout or trying a new vegetable.

3. **Stay Educated:** Monthly, read an article, research paper, or watch a documentary on health and fitness. Evolving knowledge keeps things fresh.

**Actionable Strategies for a Fit Future**

1. **Flexibility in Approach:** As life changes, so will your fitness needs. Adjust, adapt, and advance.

2. **Accountability Matters:** Share your goals with a friend or family member. Check-in with them weekly.

3. **Celebrate the Small Wins:** Every achievement, no matter how small, deserves acknowledgment.

4. **Continuous Learning:** The world of health and fitness is ever-evolving. Stay informed, and be open to trying new methods and techniques.

## A Leaf from Chris Hemsworth's Book

Hollywood actor Chris Hemsworth, known for his role as Thor, has undergone various physical transformations for his roles. From bulking up for Thor to slimming down dramatically for "In the Heart of the Sea," Chris's journey exemplifies the power of adaptability and the importance of professional guidance. His fitness app, 'Centr', embodies his belief in holistic fitness, emphasizing not just workouts but also mindfulness and nutrition. Chris's journey reminds us that fitness is multifaceted and adaptable, and with the right guidance and dedication, anything is achievable.

## **Food for Thought:** Your Personal Fitness Philosophy

Your fitness journey should echo your beliefs, goals, and lifestyle. For some, fitness might mean running marathons; for others, it's about mental well-being and maintaining a basic level of physical health. As you move forward, carve out your personal fitness philosophy. Is it about resilience? Balance? Strength? Endurance? Or is it a blend of many elements?

## Summary

Embarking on a fitness journey is one of the most empowering decisions you can make. It promises not just physical rewards but mental and emotional rejuvenation. Drawing from real-life tales, like Liam's unwavering determination or Chris Hemsworth's adaptable fitness journey, we learn that our paths will be unique but the destination is universal: a healthier, stronger version of ourselves.

Your future in fitness is bright and promising. It won't be without challenges, but armed with the knowledge from this book and an unwavering commitment to yourself, you're more than equipped to face them. Celebrate every milestone, learn from every setback, and always remember that the journey is as significant, if not more, than the destination.

As we close this chapter and this book, remember the words of the legendary runner Steve Prefontaine: "To give anything less than your best is to sacrifice the gift." You possess the incredible gift of potential; it's up to you to unleash it in your fitness journey. Embrace the road ahead, for it leads to a future where you're the healthiest and strongest version of yourself. Now, tie up those shoelaces, and let's get moving! Your future in fitness awaits.

**PS. Did this book help you in some way? If so, I'd love an honest review. That helps other readers find the right book for their needs.**